DATE		

A MODEL FOR
NATIONAL HEALTH CARE

HEALTH AND MEDICINE
IN AMERICAN SOCIETY
Series Editors
Judith Walzer Leavitt
Morris Vogel

A Model for National Health Care

THE HISTORY OF
KAISER PERMANENTE

Rickey Hendricks

RUTGERS UNIVERSITY PRESS

New Brunswick, New Jersey

Library of Congress Cataloging-in-Publication Data

Hendricks, Rickey Lynn.
    A model for national health care : the history of Kaiser
Permanente / Rickey Hendricks.
        p.   cm. — (Health and medicine in American society)
    Includes bibliographical references and index.
    ISBN 0-8135-1929-2
    1. Kaiser-Permanente Medical Care Program—History.   I. Title.
II. Series.
RA413.3.K33H46   1993
368.3'82'006573—dc20   92-29999
                                                                  CIP

British Cataloging-in-Publication information available

FOR MY DAUGHTERS

Adrienne Elizabeth Whitelaw

Abigail Kerry Whitelaw

Contents

CONTENTS

List of Tables

Preface

THIS STUDY BEGAN in the summer of 1983, which I spent in the San Francisco Bay Area doing research for a planned biography of Henry J. Kaiser—one of the first historians to gain access to the newly acquired Kaiser Papers at the Bancroft Library, University of California, Berkeley. Henry Kaiser's intensely personal involvement in the medical program bearing his name was well documented, as was his penchant for controversy and drama on the national stage. Other vital personalities involved with the health plan in its early years also appeared in the massive documentation of the industrialist's empire building from the 1930s until his death in 1967. The topic was an unmined field of inquiry in the ongoing policy debate over U.S. health care. It seemed to be a fascinating story that would contribute to knowledge about the national health care system, in economic and ethical crisis since the Medicare and Medicaid legislation of the mid-1960s.

I had a generous National Institutes of Health (NIH) grant from the National Library of Medicine for revision of a first version of this study for publication. The grant funded more research and gave me needed time to develop the topic. Other professional experiences were beneficial to my knowlege of health care and health policy from a national perspective, including work at the University of California, San Francisco. I wish to thank Dr. Norris Hundley for permission to reprint most of my article, "Medical Practice Embattled: Kaiser Permanente, the American Medical Association, and Henry J.

Kaiser on the West Coast, 1945–1955," *Pacific Historical Review* 60, no. 4 (Nov. 1991). Thanks also to the editors of the *Journal of Policy History* for allowing me to reprint segments of "Liberal Default, Labor Support, and Conservative Neutrality: The Kaiser Permanente Medical Care Program After World War II," 1, no. 2 (1989). Dr. Gert Brieger encouraged me to publish "Oral History as Social History," in the *Bulletin of the History of Medicine* 65 (1991), a review of the excellent Kaiser Permanente oral history series. The series consists of approximately twenty interviews done by Malca Chall and Sally Smith Hughes for the Bancroft Library Regional Oral History Office. The personal vignettes uncovered by Chall and Hughes enhanced my manuscript considerably.

I thank archivists and researchers for small but vital pieces of information I obtained from the International Longshoremen's and Warehousemen's Union Library, San Francisco; the United Mineworkers of America Health and Retirement Funds Archives at the University of West Virginia, Morgantown; the E. Richard Weinerman Papers at the Sterling Library, Yale University, New Haven; and the Leonard W. Larson Papers, University of North Dakota, Grand Forks. Gene Vrana of the ILWU Library and Daphna Blair, researcher at the University of West Virginia, were especially helpful.

Daniel A. Scannell, Director of Public Affairs for Kaiser Permanente, Northern California Region, and Kaiser Permanente Manager of Advertising, Donald Duffy, both showed interest in my work. They helped me obtain historical photographs and other information. I thank Dan Scannell for permission to publish the images included in this volume for the Oakland office. Other photographs are courtesy of the Bancroft Library. Drs. Cecil Cutting and Clifford H. Keene gave valuable readings to my manuscripts, as did the late Ernest Saward, for which I am most grateful. Dr. Keene has been most generous with his time and insights.

I would like to thank friends, colleagues, and family members who stood out at various critical stages in my completion of this work. I am most grateful for their patience, for their suggestions, and for their steadfast support. Colleagues who have advised and encouraged me over the years include Edward D. Berkowitz, Hamilton Cravens, Gerald N. Grob, John S. Haller, Jr., Sally Smith Hughes, and John C. Livingston. The book could not have been published without the support of Gerry Grob, Judith Walzer Leavitt, Morris J. Vogel, and Marlie Wasserman at a most critical juncture. They all have offered the best of their wisdom and expertise; none are responsible for any confusion of fact or interpretation on my part. My parents and family in Florida, Kentucky, and Colorado have given me all I have asked of them. Finally, I would like to express deep gratitude to special friends in Mill Valley who have shown me unconditional love, and how to pursue my life's work in peace and with humility. This book is dedicated to all of them as well, especially Linda Wallimann and Dick Pervier.

Introduction

HENRY J. KAISER AND SIDNEY R. GARFIELD, an industrialist and a doctor, together pioneered a medical program that changed the face of U.S. health care. In the middle third of the twentieth century, they created the world's largest private health care system, the first group health plan in the nation to fully incorporate prepayment, group practice, and substantial medical facilities on a large geographic scale.

Henry Kaiser helped turn the course of the Colorado and Columbia rivers to reclaim arid lands of the Far West during the Great Depression. He completed large federal contracts on the major New Deal dams of the 1930s: Hoover on the Nevada-Arizona border, Grand Coulee and Bonneville in Washington, and Shasta in California. In 1938 southern California physician Sidney Garfield set up a medical program under contract with the Kaiser company for about 5,000 workers at Grand Coulee Dam in eastern Washington. During World War II, the two men joined forces again at Kaiser's shipyards on the West Coast at Richmond in northern California, and at Portland-Vancouver in Oregon and Washington. Garfield established the shipyard medical programs for Kaiser's work force of 200,000, as well as a much smaller one for 3,000 steelworkers at the Kaiser Fontana plant east of Los Angeles.

The company formed the Permanente and the Northern Permanente foundations as charitable trusts in 1942 to support the health plan and medical facilities at these three sites. In mid-1945 former workers and AFL-CIO unions in the region prompted the trustees to take the health program beyond Kaiser plant gates to the surrounding communities. After World War II the Kaiser Permanente Health Plan, a nonprofit trust, developed separately from Kaiser industries. It dwindled temporarily to a few thousand after the shipyards closed, but membership reached 524,000 within a decade.[1]

By 1970 Kaiser Permanente had 2.1 million members and began to expand eastward. It was the largest, most integrated, and most expansive of the nation's prepaid group health plans, redefined as "health maintenance organizations" in the federal HMO Act of 1973.[2] By 1990, as the largest HMO in the nation, Kaiser Permanente had twelve regions nationwide with over 6.5 million members, 7,760 physicians, over 7,000 licensed beds, and total assets of $4.9 billion. It had 2.4 million members in northern California, almost a third of the regional population. The press reported that Kaiser was 30%– 50% lower in price than most indemnity plans, and 10%–20% lower than other HMOs. It will end the twentieth century with about a $10 billion capital spending plan in California.[3]

Kaiser Permanente both absorbed and produced the shock waves of vast socioeconomic change in the Pacific West during the 1930s and the 1940s. It was a regional response to temporal, geophysical, and demographic conditions. It became a national model for reshaping the structure of U.S. health care. As a free enterprise alternative to national health insurance and socialized medicine perpetually rejected by the nation's policymakers, Kaiser Permanente was a prototype for health care reform within the limits of U.S. politics and liberal economics, a masterpiece of ideological ambiguity and political consensus.

The term *health maintenance* had a dual genesis in public health and industrial medicine. It was predicated on preventive medicine and broad access to comprehensive care for blue- and white-collar workers and their families. In 1920 Yale professor of public health C.-E.A. Winslow defined public health practice as "the education of the individual in principles of personal hygiene, the organization of medical and nursing service for the early diagnosis and preventive treatment of disease, and the development of the social machinery which will ensure to every individual a standard of living adequate for the maintenance of health."[4]

In a 1945 *Fortune* magazine article, Garfield stated that "maintenance of health" was the central mission of the Kaiser program.[5] Three functional principles shaped the program's development in its first two decades: prepayment through the Kaiser Foundation Health Plans, Inc., group practice in the Permanente Medical Groups, and complete facilities supported by Kaiser Foundation Hospitals, Inc. These principles shaped the program in its contemporary form during corporate reorganization in the late 1950s. At a meeting in early March 1970 at the Kaiser building in Oakland, health plan executive counsel Scott Fleming met with Paul M. Ellwood, Jr., M.D., health policy adviser to the Nixon administration. They drafted a "conceptual outline" for a bill to legitimize and give federal support to prepaid corporate plans like Kaiser Permanente, as yet unnamed. They adjourned to a Mexican restaurant where they discussed the term *HMO* over a pitcher of margaritas.[6]

Three circumstances framed early development of the Kaiser Permanente program: its regional character, the collective identity that evolved among plan physicians, and the recognition of the mutual benefits of prepaid group medicine. Kaiser Permanente was the product of the geophysical, socioeconomic, and political environment of the Pacific West—its rugged natural resource and maritime industries, volatile population, and aggressive union movement—as well as of the creative impulses of Kaiser and Garfield. Its membership mirrored the restless working-class population that migrated to the western water projects and maritime industries during the depression and World War II in California, Oregon, and Washington.

The California population grew by 20 percent during the depression, and a third again from 1940 to 1950. Federal spending in the state rose to nearly $35 billion. Kaiser's mammoth government reclamation and shipbuilding contracts added significantly to the socioeconomic shock waves that hit the region.[7] Franklin D. Roosevelt's New Deal labor policy spurred union growth, solidarity, and welfare demands. The

1935 National Labor Relations Act legitimized industrial unionism under John L. Lewis and the Congress of Industrial Organizations (CIO). Union membership tripled from 1933 to 1938, as militancy erupted. In California the left-wing long-shoremen, led by the fiery Harry Bridges, shut down the San Francisco waterfront twice during the decade. Bridges and Lewis both played a part in giving national visibility to Kaiser's health program, as aggressive West Coast union locals compelled its expansion after World War II.[8]

Early Permanente physician leaders also fit a regional character cast. Like nineteenth-century pioneers willing to risk all for the main chance, physicians flocked to the West from centers of medical progressivism in other regions for the healthful environment and in hopes of striking it rich. By the early 1900s San Francisco was regarded as "the most heavily hospital-bedded city in the nation," attended by a high concentration of physicians with incomes comparable to those of skilled laborers. Unfavorable professional demographics persisted through the century.[9] This poor economic outlook prompted doctors with an entrepreneurial drive or a public health orientation to leave independent fee-for-service practice to join the Permanente physicians' group.

The perspective of Garfield and his associates contrasted with the elite scientific view that biomedical research and new technology were the keys to limitless improvement of the human condition.[10] They sought broad patient access to preventive, holistic care to improve the quality of ordinary lives.

The Permanente physicians survived demoralizing collegial conflict and clashes with Henry Kaiser by creating their own medical practice culture. It germinated at Grand Coulee Dam and developed at the Pacific Coast shipyards, where group physicians were protected from outside detractors by the cocoon of Kaiser resources and facilities. Group identity had the same meaning for the doctors that union membership had for their patients. It gave them the strength to assert collective authority within the corporate power structure, as well as to withstand the condemnation of their outside colleagues. The Permanente physicians thus played out early what would become the core crisis of their profession over the second half of

the twentieth century. The rapid expansion of Kaiser Permanente at mid-century heralded a decisive shift in U.S. medicine away from solo fee-for-service practice to the prepaid
group plans and health maintenance organizations (HMOs)
that transformed the structure of the country's health care.[11]

Kaiser Permanente emerged from the New Deal and wartime partnership of industry, labor, and government among
several hundred group prepayment plans organized by private industry, small private physicians' groups, and consumer
cooperatives. Kaiser was the largest of these plans, but it
shared characteristics with smaller plans on both the Atlantic
and Pacific coasts. In contrast to the paternalism of European
medicine replicated in early U.S. hospitals on the eastern sea-
board, prepaid group plans in the United States were voluntary and egalitarian.[12] They clustered on the urban coast and
in regions with large numbers of workers in natural resource
industries at isolated sites. The earliest plans dated to the California gold rush in 1849, and to construction of the transcontinental railroad in the 1860s. Workers and entrepreneurs
who migrated west left familiar community welfare networks
and were compelled to create new ones. In so doing, they rejected traditional dependency and class control in capital-
labor relations as well as the paternalism and deference that
separated doctor and patient.

The first prepaid group program in the nation was the compulsory federal Marine Hospital Service, established in 1798
as a means for communities to contain communicable diseases
spread by the transient seafaring labor force. The marine
service became the U.S. Public Health Service (PHS) in 1912.[13]
The first commercial insurance company also emerged from
maritime culture. The Massachusetts Health Insurance Company of Boston was incorporated in 1847, at the same time the
American Medical Association (AMA) was formed in New
York state. The State Marine Hospital was established in San
Francisco the first year of the gold rush. The earliest voluntary, private, prepaid group plan in the nation also appeared
in the volatile port city. The first was La Société Française de
Bienfaisance Mutuelle, established by the San Francisco
French community the first year of the gold rush. La Société

was followed by formation of other ethnic and fraternal group plans across the bay from Kaiser's Oakland headquarters in the next century. The Southern Pacific Railroad Company established a health plan in 1868, the oldest large industrial prepayment plan to survive into the twentieth century.[14]

At the turn of the century, physicians in Oregon and Washington willing to follow the work force entered contract practice in large numbers in the railroad, lumber, and mining industries. Workers' compensation laws encouraged expansion of industrial plans. Between 1910 and 1920 the Pacific states were first with these laws. By 1917 the *Report of the Social Insurance Commission* indicated that a third of all lower and middle income wage earners in California were covered by a variety of cash indemnity "sickness" plans and contract medical care.[15]

The Western Federation of Miners (WFM) established a large mutual aid and hospital network that accounted for a large number of the hospital beds in the West. Historians claim that care of the sick moved from home to hospital most rapidly in the western mining states. By 1920 a number of the leading states in per capita supply of hospital beds were in the western hardrock mining regions. Hospital death rates are one measure of rising reliance on hospital care, even in terminal cases. In the mid-1930s over a fourth of U.S. deaths were in hospitals; by 1940, nearly a third. At the height of peak wartime mobilization on the West Coast in 1943, more than 45 percent of all deaths in California and Washington were in hospitals, as well as in the mining states of Colorado, Montana, Nevada, and Wyoming.[16]

Doctors in the West established a larger proportion of proprietary medical institutions than those in other regions of the nation, including the proprietary medical schools and hospitals that were forebears of the University of California, San Francisco and the Stanford University medical centers. By 1923 an AMA study reported that 52 percent of hospitals in the Pacific states were proprietary, and only 12 percent were municipal or voluntary. By contrast, those of the Mid-Atlantic were 49 percent voluntary, and only 17 percent proprietary.[17]

The urban coast also fostered large state and municipal employee group plans that emerged from the New Deal. They had a wide range of working agreements with doctors. The Ross-Loos Clinic was created by a private group practice in Los Angeles in 1929 for several thousand municipal water board employees. The Health Service System began for city workers in San Francisco in 1938. Within a decade 900 local independent doctors who had agreed to serve members under a loose reimbursement plan were disgruntled and resigned. Members joined Kaiser. Federal bureaucrats of the Home Owner's Loan Corporation in Washington, D.C., established the Group Health Association (GHA) in 1937. By 1938 membership was over 6,000. Full-time doctors were salaried by the lay consumer–controlled board of directors.[18]

Almost immediately, the cooperative was forced into court to protect its physicians from discrimination by the AMA-affiliated local medical society. The District of Columbia Medical Society (DCMS), backed by the AMA, threatened GHA physicians with expulsion from the society for "unethical conduct"; one doctor was expelled. He therefore lost his malpractice insurance and was denied privileges by hospitals afraid of losing AMA approval. In some local hospitals GHA physicians were not allowed to attend their emergency patients. The Justice Department prosecuted the AMA, DCMS, and twenty-one physicians for restraint of trade.[19] Despite escalating AMA opposition, World War II made prepaid group practice increasingly popular as military doctors and civilian war personnel shared cooperative experiences.[20]

After his wartime shipyards sharply curtailed production, Henry Kaiser's self-contained medical edifice still towered over the San Francisco Bay Area landscape surrounding his corporate headquarters. Kaiser was a master of the dramatic construction feat and the media event in health care as in industry. He moved between epic and melodrama, from gargantuan acts of creation to petty conflicts with associates, including physicians, whom he often offended with his bullish manner. His company's transition from industrial to general community health care after World War II paralleled its diversification to domestic construction and manufacturing, in aluminum, steel, homes, and automobiles for the white- and blue-collar consumer. Sharing in a national planning spirit at the end of the war, the popular industrialist presented the program as the model for a national health plan in the nation's capital and the press. In a sense the Kaiser plan was a diffuse form of his self-contained company dam and ship-building communities. Kaiser's expansiveness and national vision alarmed the majority of independent fee-for-service physicians, represented by the AMA, which opposed Kaiser Permanente over succeeding decades to little avail.

Large government and union groups eagerly joined Kaiser and other new plans. In 1947 Kaiser acquired the 19,000 municipal employees in San Francisco from the Health Service System. The Health Insurance Plan of New York (HIP) incorporated the same year for a projected 150,000 city employees under the leadership of Mayor Fiorello LaGuardia. Second only to Kaiser in membership, HIP did not have facilities or a fully committed medical group. The United Mine Workers (UMW) Health and Retirement Funds formed in 1947, with over 85 percent of union members using group prepayment plans. Like GHA, the UMW health program headquartered in Washington, D.C. The UMW likewise differed from Kaiser. Fund managers paid physicians and hospitals independently for care of union members.[21]

AMA doctors continued to oppose flagrant expansion of these plans into their professional domain. They feared loss of control over medical practice, as well as economic competition. They believed their cultural identity and income depended on the personal doctor-patient relationship, bonded by direct payment for care.[22] AMA action against the general spread of unorthodox plans surfaced with the depression. In the early 1930s practitioners' incomes plummeted because patients could not afford private fees.[23] Physicians in San Francisco suffered added distress. The California Medical Economic Survey reported in 1934 that the net median income of city physicians in 1933, the trough of the depression, was $2,300, fallen from $6,000 in 1929. Membership in the county medical society declined 18 percent because doctors could not afford dues. Thus the profession lost leverage over standards of practice. Nevertheless, the physician population in the city increased by 12 percent from 1934 to 1940, and by 30 percent more during the 1940s.[24]

National health politics in the 1940s increased doctors' economic and status anxiety. The year 1943 was a political Armageddon for the AMA. Senator Robert Wagner of New York spearheaded a series of compulsory national health insurance bills from 1943 to 1947.[25] Wagner's name also appeared on the National Labor Relations Act of 1935. The connection between suspected Communist influence in the labor movement and socialized medicine was not lost on Republican and AMA conservatives. In confrontation with New Deal Democrats over national health, the AMA seemed to gather its varied opponents onto a single battleground. The first Wagner bill appeared the year of peak wartime mobilization. East Coast politicians such as Mayor LaGuardia of New York, Senator Wagner, and Florida's Claude Pepper treated Kaiser as an instant expert on the nation's health because of the high visibility of his shipyard health plan. A landmark 1943 U.S. Supreme Court decision upheld a lower court finding against the AMA and local medical society doctors for denying GHA doctors society membership. The decision validated principles of free trade and competition in medical reform. It cast medical practice as a "trade," challenging ancient shibboleths regarding the mystical doctor-patient trust and the physician's venerable status in U.S. culture.[26]

Newly powerful CIO unionists also opposed the AMA. They supported Kaiser's medical program as an alternative to national insurance proposals, perennially buried in congressional committee. Harry Bridges led the International Longshoremen's and Warehousemen's Union (ILWU) to join Kaiser Permanente in 1950, in a Pacific coastwide contract. The same year Bridges's union was ousted from the CIO for alleged Communist ties. The lionlike UMW president John L. Lewis also wanted Kaiser for his members in the early 1950s. Garfield tried to establish a plan in the Southeast at Lewis's behest, though the idea quickly fizzled. The CIO union connections drew political attention to Permanente physicians for suspected Communist activities at Vallejo, California, where they treated UMW members for neuromuscular injury and disease.

Henry Kaiser made relations with the doctors worse by attempting his own anticommunist purge. In a parody of McCarthy-era witch hunts, Kaiser devised a loyalty oath for the physicians and staff to deter FBI scrutiny, alienating health plan physicians. At the same time he ordered his own name placed on the health plan and hospitals, to replace the Permanente Foundation title. Permanente doctors rebelled against corporate authority, retaining "Permanente" for the medical group.

The separate name did not give the group an independent identity. They still suffered the Kaiser stigma among their local colleagues, who despised Henry Kaiser's public prominence. The fast growth of the health plan and hospitals, strong labor ties, and attraction of large government employee groups escalated anxiety over status and income among local medical societies.[27] Kaiser made it worse by bombastic potshots and threats of litigation against them.

Permanente doctors were the scapegoats for the unwelcome trend toward prepaid group practice in their profession. They were a highly visible target. By 1955 there were 500 Permanente doctors at a time when only about 5 percent of U.S. doctors were engaged in any kind of group practice. In turmoil themselves, they did not appreciate their pioneering role. Internal stresses between Kaiser and the doctors nearly shattered Kaiser Permanente at its peak of expansion at midcentury. This history of the company's first two decades is a story of bold individuals who made a dramatic impact on the contemporary shape of U.S. medicine and health.

1   Reclamation and Health in the Arid West

Born in upstate New York in 1882, Henry Kaiser migrated West as a young man in 1906. His first company was Kaiser Paving, established in British Columbia in 1914 for the modest purpose of paving city streets in Vancouver and Nainamo. The U.S. automobile culture drew the nascent industrialist back across the border to build roads and irrigation projects in sparsely populated parts of the West.

Kaiser family life was transient. The contractor, his wife, and his sons often slept in the open, in tents, and in cars along with the crews. His mobile household and office saved Kaiser much time and money as he shuttled from project to project. Also, the vagabond existence enhanced the camaraderie and easy physical contact with workers. He became familiar with medical needs in Washington and other western states as he searched for doctors in the nearest towns to treat injured workers.[1] The mobility and rootlessness of the Kaiser family reflected the character of the regional population.

Kaiser balanced his own weak tie to geographic place with a strong sense of the elemental components of community in newly developing areas. He was instinctively a regionalist who saw the interplay of geography, demography, and natural resource industries as the generating dynamic of social change and economic growth. Kaiser had abandoned formal education at age thirteen; he was not an intellectual and would have ignored work by Lewis Mumford, Patrick Geddes, and other theorists of the Regional Planning Association of America in the 1920s. Regionalists, Mumford wrote, attempt "to utilize, rather than to nullify or destroy, [a region's] natural advantages." They see "people, industry and the land as a single unit." When Kaiser developed the industrial sites where his health plan began in the 1930s and early 1940s, however, he mirrored such theorists' recommendations.[2]

In March 1931 Kaiser and other members of the Six Companies consortium he had joined to bid on New Deal reclamation projects won a $48.9 million contract with the federal government to build Hoover Dam in the arid Southwest. In 1938 the Kaiser company began another construction contract at Grand Coulee Dam in eastern Washington state. Franklin D. Roosevelt's administration sought to expand the arable land base and public power in the Far West. The dams also served FDR's New Deal as a public relations project, an example of a new conquest of the wilderness, that might renew the frontier spirit in the public imagination and offer hope to the nation's fifteen million unemployed.[3] The dams also gave Henry Kaiser national visibility and bold, heroic stature. They schooled the industrialist in government and labor relations and set the stage for innovation in industrial medicine.

At Desert Center on the Los Angeles Aqueduct in southern California, and at Grand Coulee Dam in east central Washington, physician Sidney R. Garfield integrated prepayment, group practice, and clinical facilities to provide comprehensive care for workers. At these sites, Garfield and his physician associates enacted a creation myth of corporate medical culture. Their shared values and experiences on the water projects in the arid West would carry them through the first quarter-century of trial and conflict as the Kaiser medical program developed.

Garfield was not the first in the field of contract practice and prepaid group health, which were common in the natural resource industries of the Far West. Huge reclamation projects to bring water and power to burgeoning Los Angeles County in southern California and to other Pacific states stimulated innovation among doctors, laborers, and employers at desolate labor sites. In 1908 young Raymond G. Taylor completed an internship at Los Angeles County Hospital and signed a contract as physician-in-chief with the Los Angeles Board of Public Works to "undertake the organization, equipment, and administration" of a medical department to care for 10,000 workers during the construction of the Los Angeles Aqueduct running from Haiwee Dam. Aqueduct workers paid a dollar a month assessment if their monthly wage was forty dollars, and fifty cents if it was lower.

Taylor provided all medical care "except for venereal disease, intemperance, vicious habits, injuries received in fights, or chronic diseases acquired before employment." The city built field hospitals with beds for six patients. Those able to travel were taken to Los Angeles General Hospital by wagon and railroad. In addition to two partners, Dr. Taylor employed other physicians, hospital stewards, and nurses, who also received room and board. The contract ended in 1913 with quite a handsome gross return of almost $164,000.[4]

Contract doctors served a unique working-class culture that evolved in western resource industries. Massive technology increased risks of spectacular accidents. Mining was a deadly occupation in the Southeast and the West, and the Western Federation of Miners and United Mine Workers pioneered in creating health and mutual welfare networks throughout their farflung work environment. Welfare unionism was a community-building influence in regional working-class society. At the New Deal dams, Henry Kaiser added the element of expansive welfare capitalism, prompted by early passage of state worker's compensation laws in California and Washington in 1911, and by 1913 in twenty-three other states.[5]

The AMA condemned contract practice, even as the trend grew in the region. AMA and labor leaders both charged that company-paid doctors were unsympathetic to patients and represented employer "intrusion . . . into intimate family relationships." Company doctors had complete access to patient records, they claimed, and thus threatened family economic survival. The AMA attacked this practice on ethical as well as humanitarian grounds. It was "virtually impossible to hold a corporation responsible for the maintenance of standards of practice."[6] The AMA vehemently defended the traditional system of solo fee-for-service practice because it preserved values of individualism, voluntarism, and the doctor-patient trust. Direct payment for care signified this trust, giving both participants a stake in the healing process.[7] Despite AMA disapproval, economically strapped doctors continued to accept industrial labor contracts and entered other unorthodox forms of practice. These proliferated in progressive coastal cities as well as in rural and agricultural regions.

The depression brought a national average decline in physicians' income of 17 percent. Doctors in farming regions suffered declines as great as 50 percent. By 1932 at least 27 percent of Washington State physicians, and probably many more, were employed under contracts, mostly serving industrial workers. In farming regions doctors entered prepayment agreements with the Farm Security Administration (FSA) farmer cooperatives. Because illness and disability were the primary reasons for default of government relief loans, the agency formed medical cooperatives among more than 600,000 farm families in one-third of the nation's rural counties.[8] The FSA cooperatives were thus founded to protect government loans rather than as an effort in national medical planning.

The Committee on the Costs of Medical Care (CCMC), in existence from 1927 to 1932, was the single organized effort at national health planning to address the widespread medical indigency of the era. Recognizing the deplorable health conditions suffered by indigent and working-class Americans, as well as the precarious income of independent physicians, the committee majority recommended national reform through regional group practice associations and community medical centers. The centers would disseminate knowledge downward to local doctors, clinics, and hospitals. The CCMC was largely ineffective. Its critique of independent fee-for-service practice alienated traditional practitioners, who represented the majority of the profession.

The committee reported that "many of the practitioners who work alone are unable to afford the costly and varied equipment necessary for diagnosing and treating all illnesses; nor do they have the time to become proficient in its use." The report noted that salaried physicians had a higher average income than general practitioners in private practice. It adopted the language of industrial efficiency, reducing the patient to a natural resource, "wasted" if not well maintained. The committee also criticized the inefficient separation of medical service and hospitalization, complaining that facilities were "duplicated" between hospitals and doctors' offices and were "insufficiently utilized in both." Beds were empty, while physicians, dentists, and nurses stood "idle." Nevertheless, many patients suffered and died due to inattention.[9]

Although their mandate was to reduce cost and improve access to clinical care, the CCMC reformers appeared to focus on elite intellectual resources. The majority advocated a regional distribution of research and education centers, a structure that Daniel Fox labels "hierarchical regionalism." The scientific elite would redistribute new knowledge and expert training downward to the level of basic care by small-town physicians.[10] Eight of the nine physicians serving on the CCMC took issue with the majority, warning in a minority report that the committee recommendations were "suggestive of the great mergers in industry, the main medical center being in the nature of the parent holding company . . . the adoption by medicine of the technique of big business, that is, mass production."[11]

Like other national planning theories of the era, the CCMC recommendations had little practical effect. Pragmatists in industry, the labor movement, and the prepaid group health movement initiated private sector plans on an ad hoc basis, with no centralized planning. Yet the committee recommendations had two lasting effects. More than a decade after the final CCMC report, the committee view was reflected in the elaborate government and philanthropic funding structure that materialized after World War II.[12] The second effect of the CCMC reports was to polarize the U.S. medical community. The report accentuated the dichotomy between liberals and the conservative grass roots of the profession, establishing a rhetoric for conflict that far outlasted memory of the CCMC report. Traditional doctors reacted against the broad socio-economic trends that undermined solo practice, changing the shape of the twentieth-century U.S. hospital from a charitable institution to an impersonal bureaucratic model that doctors feared. Sociologist Talcott Parsons later provided the classic argument that they reacted to modern trends by clinging to the idea of doctor-patient trust, signified by the personal exchange between them of direct payment for care as the last vestige of traditional small-town practice.[13]

Reform came from the base of the national medical care pyramid, from patients, consumers, and unorthodox practioners, rather than from the elite of the medical profession. In 1929 the stock market crash signaled the onset of the Great Depression, and three types of group prepayment plans appeared to challenge independent fee-for-service practice. They were organically rooted in the dynamic material culture of the blue- and white-collar workers whom they served. All appeared west of the Mississippi River, on the urban coast or in inland regions with economies dependent upon natural resources. They served large urban employee groups accustomed to collective action, and rural groups in regions with consumer cooperative traditions dating from the early twentieth century.

In Dallas, Texas, a group of about 1,500 teachers paid fifty cents a month to join a hospitalization plan at Baylor University Hospital begun in 1929. A year later seven hospitals in Sacramento, California, set up an insurance company to administer a similar plan. Other plans sprang up in Grinnell, Iowa, and Rockford, Illinois. Before 1936 fifteen hospital prepayment plans existed in eleven states, forming the Blue Cross network. By 1940 Blue Cross covered half the insured individuals in the country.[14] Doctors accepted the concept of hospitalization insurance because it separated the practice of medicine from the "workshops" and "tools" of the profession.

In the Midwest, Dr. Michael Shadid of Elk City, Oklahoma, started a consumer cooperative for local farmers over the objections of the local medical society affiliate of the AMA. Only with the support of the populist Oklahoma Farmers' Union did Shadid obtain a loan to build a hospital. The county medical society did not wish to risk litigation by expelling Shadid, so its membership dissolved and then reformed a year and a half later, excluding him. Geographic isolation and the support of the farmers' union enabled the cooperative to survive, but Shadid faced continual difficulties with licensing and other collegial authority wielded by the society, hampering his employment of good physicians.[15]

The Los Angeles County Medical Association (LACMA) made a bolder assault on a local prepaid group practice plan, also begun in 1929. Drs. Donald Ross and H. Clifford Loos established the Ross-Loos Clinic to serve 2,000 members of the Los Angeles County Employees Association of the Department of Water and Power. By the mid-1930s a group of about fifty doctors served approximately 40,000 people. Average total payments by individual subscribers averaged $2.69 a family per month. Services included comprehensive office and hospital care, diagnostic testing, surgery, ambulance, and other services for half the fee-for-service cost reported by a California State Emergency Relief Agency survey for urban family care.[16]

The Ross-Loos departure from solo fee-for-service practice alarmed local doctors now faced with hard economic times. Drs. Ross and Loos literally were cast out of the professional fraternity in more than the biblical sense. They ate of the forbidden fruit of enterprise and experiment at a time when the profession was in no mood for deviant behavior. In February 1934 they were notified to appear before the LACMA Board of Councilors in ten days "to show cause" why they "should not be censored and/or suspended, and/or expelled." Contrary to the rules of U.S. jurisprudence, they were guilty until proven innocent of unspecified charges. They learned through a telephone inquiry that the charge was unethical advertising. Although they produced substantial evidence that they had not paid solicitors or for literature aimed at recruiting subscribers, the local association voted unanimously for expulsion. The California Medical Association (CMA) concurred without dissent, but the action was rejected by the

AMA Judicial Council on technical grounds. The association ruled that procedural irregularities, not the merits of the case, made the local society judgment invalid.

In a later report the AMA nevertheless alluded to the clinic group as if it was unethically financed. Allegedly, 1933 and 1934 receipts from soda fountain, magazine, and candy sales amounted to well over $18,000 and were vital to the clinic's solvency. "Apparently it is necessary for the Ross-Loos Medical Group," the report stated, "to rely on fees from dependents who are not included on the monthly prepayment insurance basis." It went on to state that although clinics organized by private physicians' groups were "less undesirable than those organized by individual promoters," the participation of Ross and Loos in "contract practice arrangements" with employee groups offset this dubious advantage in the perception of the professional judiciary.[17] The stigma of their attempted expulsion lingered on.

Since the real authority of the AMA was at the local level, the Ross-Loos physicians were, in effect, ostracized by their professional colleagues. The legal right to practice medicine was not contingent on membership in the county medical society, but doctors who were not members remained outside the professional referral network, were denied hospital privileges, and were unable to take specialty board examinations that became more important as specialization increased in the following decade. Despite their pariah status medical innovators continued to find the southern California desert fertile ground for contracts in the large-scale natural resource industries of the 1930s.

The group prepayment plans and the FSA medical cooperatives of the 1930s were geographically scattered and served a minuscule portion of the medically needy population. In 1930 only an estimated one million U.S. workers were covered by prepaid medical service plans, jointly sponsored by employers, out of a total labor force of 48.8 million. Groups covered were small and occupationally specific. More than half of the plan members were employed in the dangerous and isolated natural resource industries as miners and lumber workers. They included 540,000 people in twenty-one states.[18] Because of the physician surplus, the strength of the labor

movement, and the influence of large-scale resource industries in the region, physicians in Oregon and Washington continued to enter contract practice in large numbers. In 1932, 80
percent said that it prevailed in their communities.[19]

The big reclamation projects brought more workers to the
arid West in the 1930s, including young Dr. Sidney Garfield.
After he graduated from the University of Iowa Medical
School, Garfield returned to his hometown of Los Angeles,
whose county population grew by well over half a million in
the 1930s. During the week the young physician was what colleagues called "super resident on surgery" at the 3,000-bed
Los Angeles County Hospital, which served the city's indigent.
It and the public hospital at Tulane were the largest in the
country. Fellow physicians Raymond Kay and Morris Collen
served under Garfield's supervision.[20]

The experience of Garfield, Kay, and Collen at the Los Angeles County Hospital acquainted the young doctors with the
collegial benefits of group practice in a large urban setting.
Their preference was unusual at a time when there were well
under 2,000 group practitioners in the United States. A large
number of these were with the Mayo Clinic in Rochester, Minnesota, the first large group practice in the nation, and within
the regional orb of Garfield's medical education, as well as that
of several of his midwestern colleagues, including Collen. Garfield spoke on occasion of establishing a "little Mayo Clinic" in
California.

Times were uncertain for young physicians, and incomes
precarious. Between 1929 and 1932 the CCMC reported that
one-third of all private practitioners had net incomes of less
than $2,300. From the late 1920s until the early 1950s emer-
gency hospital surgeons in San Francisco usually earned less
than electrical line workers, plumbers, and fire captains.[21]

Faced with opening a private practice in the midst of the
depression, supplemented by a part-time teaching position at
the University of Southern California Medical School, Garfield chose instead to begin an isolated industrial medical
practice in the Mojave Desert.

Garfield went to work on the Los Angeles Aqueduct running from Parker Dam, and then to the Grand Coulee Dam
project in east central Washington. In 1933 he contracted with

Industrial Indemnity, an insurance consortium formed by big construction contractors in the 1920s, including Henry J. Kaiser, and used in the 1930s by the companies involved in the Colorado River and Hoover Dam projects to comply with the workers' compensation law. Garfield's association with Henry Kaiser would continue until Kaiser's death in 1967.

Garfield conducted his contract practice from a small town called Desert Center, midway along the 190-mile Colorado River Aqueduct running from Parker Dam to the outskirts of Los Angeles. His charge was medical care of 5,000 "medically neglected" men, spread out over the extent of the aqueduct.[22] The decision to go out into the desert first seemed a retreat from the modern practice of Garfield's experience but offered several important advantages, psychological and practical. The desert was a tabula rasa, free from the scrutiny of a local medical establishment. Even the minority dissenters to the CCMC proposal for community-based group practice admitted the existence of special circumstances at remote labor sites.[23] The extent of contract practice in the Far West that had long operated outside the circumference of AMA activity in urban areas also insulated Garfield from criticism by his peers. Just as the California gold rush attracted migrant doctors to seek their fortunes, the aggressive labor movement and lucrative New Deal contracts now drew adventuresome physicians to remote labor sites during the hard times of the Great Depression.

At the same time, the early phases of union organizing at the reclamation sites were a proving ground in labor relations for Henry Kaiser and his fellow contractors on the big federal dam projects. Physical occupational risks at the Kaiser projects increased the workers' sense of community and union loyalty. Cases of death and disability were common in the work experience of Kaiser dam builders in the 1930s. Just before passage of state workers' compensation, accidents caused over 23 percent of all coal miners' deaths, 72 percent of deaths among powder makers, and well over 46 percent among electrical line workers. The dramatic hazards associated with mining and hardrock drilling—electricity, blasting, and rail transportation—were present on a spectacular scale at the Kaiser dams at Hoover and Grand Coulee.[24]

The Hoover Dam site, about thirty miles south of Las Vegas, Nevada, at the Black Canyon of the Colorado River, was described by journalist Theodore White as "a deadly desert place." As construction began, over a thousand transient workers and their families clustered in a "Ragtown" built of scraps of lumber, rags, tar paper, and cardboard cartons. They hoped for work that would pay four to ten dollars a day.[25]

In the spring of 1931 excavation of the access roads and a railroad bed into the Black Canyon caused the first injuries and death. A dynamite charge blew one miner fifty feet onto a rock, causing a severe back injury. Within two weeks a couple of workers were swept to the canyon bottom from the Arizona cliff face, crushed beyond recognition. Nevertheless, Six Companies directors and Bureau of Reclamation Commissioner Elwood Meade praised construction supervisor F. T. Crowe for his speed. Six Companies faced a $3,000-a-day fine if the contractor failed to divert the Colorado River's flow by 1 October 1933.

Crowe's tight schedule added to the danger and stress to the workers. In the spring and summer months men worked full shifts with temperatures of 119 degrees in the shade, and as high as 140 degrees in the airless, carbon monoxide–filled shafts. The white-hot heat impaired the workers' motor abilities, judgment, and spirits, and accidents were frequent, as were cases of temporary insanity, family abuse, and violence. Icy water splashed on the victim in his tent by co-workers was the only medical service rendered at the site for the convulsions and vomiting of heat prostration. A steady stream of heat-stricken men was transported to the hospital in Las Vegas an hour away. Sixteen died. One doctor reported that some of the prostrated dam workers had body temperatures as high as 112 degrees.

Living quarters posed a less dramatic but more general health hazard. Barracks perched on a steep mountainside housed 480 men in 1931. They had no showers, electricity, or cooling equipment. Drinking water pumped from the Colorado River was stored in huge open tanks, where bacteria causing dysentery bred and where the hot metal-heated water was undrinkable. Open outdoor toilets swarmed with flies and filled the air with the stench of disinfectant and men's physical disorders.[26]

Thousands of applicants migrated to the remote site out of economic desperation, and over 20,000 more applicants than jobs were listed on the employment rolls. Yet workers were regaining political power. National politicians and some industrialists sought to bolster union strength as a foundation for rebuilding the crumbled economy. Company improvements such as installation of a water cooler and the transport of artesian well water from Las Vegas into the work camps were a response to federal health and safety requirements. Blasting material was moved away from the machine shops.

The dam project became a stage for radical union activity. After the right-wing backlash against militant unionism in 1919, the Big Red Scare, the Industrial Workers of the World (IWW) had diminished to a small core. Now the press reported renewed IWW organizing against Six Companies led by Frank Anderson and his cohorts from their headquarters in Las Vegas. They publicized the contractors' violations of Nevada and Arizona mining and safety laws, the reckless speedup, and deplorable living conditions at the dam site. Six Companies, the Bureau of Reclamation, and Las Vegas town officials sought the arrest and jailing of unionists on various charges in June and July 1931; by mid-July, they were freed and resumed recruitment and newspaper sales, but harassment by local officials continued.[27]

The parching and hallucinogenic heat was beyond company control. Heat prostration struck several men a day in July and August, and several women collapsed and died of the heat in Ragtown. Six Companies ignited the simmering anger and frustration of dam workers on August 7 when it announced a wage cut for several dozen unskilled diversion tunnel workers; the men went on strike.[28] The company reported that only one-fourth of the work crew of 2,800 was involved in the strike, and that extreme heat was the main cause of medical problems and discontent among workers. Also the company attributed the prostration to a poor preemployment diet of coffee and donuts followed by overeating from the unlimited food provided at the mess hall for the daily room, board, and transportation fee of $1.60. Even the independent press reported that hungry men gorged themselves—one to death—on the sudden abundance of food.

The prolabor press reported a walkout of half rather than a quarter of the work force in August 1931 and identified the danger involved in the work, rather than the heat, as the cause of unrest. Men scaled vertical canyon walls almost 1,000 feet high "hanging from ropes and wire ladders." Dynamite was in constant use. Loose and falling rock was a constant menace for those scaling the cliff faces and those in the suffocating heat below on the canyon floor. Supervisor Crowe was accused of strong-arm tactics. "The company moved in a small arsenal," one source reported, "including shot-guns, rifles, teargas, guns, etc., and deputized a crew of company gunmen." U.S. government representatives entered the federal dam reservation, allegedly at labor's request. Violent confrontation between striking workers and armed strikebreakers sent in by Six Companies was averted by the timely arrival of U.S. marshals. The awesome display of state and federal enforcement officials defused the standoff, and the 1,200 strikers still on the reservation left peaceably. The strike ended eight days after it began.[29]

In the summer of 1932 a team of Harvard physiologists reported that dehydration, not overeating, caused heat prostration.[30] Moreover, most medical problems in the first year of the dam project were caused by tunneling, poor tool and material handling, falling rock, flying objects, falls, strains, and sprains.[31] Added to the daily dangers of cave-ins, dynamite blasts, high voltage lines, and falls, was the toxic mixture inside the diversion tunnels of carbon monoxide, gasoline fumes, and dust. Tunnel workers with respiratory problems that resulted from the toxic air were diagnosed at the twenty-bed company hospital with pneumonia or influenza. This was the subject of dark humor among the workers: "Up there a fellow always died of pneumonia," one quipped, "never of anything else."[32]

According to one historian, Six Companies directors protected their $300,000 investment in gasoline-fueled trucks against threats of litigation. They kept the project moving ahead rapidly, rather than install electric motors. In the summer and fall of 1933 six civil suits were filed in Nevada district court by former Six Companies workers alleging violation of Nevada mining safety laws. Each sought $75,000 in damages plus back pay for permanent disability.

Success in even one "gas case" could mean disaster for the company; more than 1,000 men had worked the tunnels, with hundreds currently employed there. San Francisco attorney Paul Marrin of Thelen and Marrin, who remained with Kaiser throughout the early decades of health plan formation, sought to discredit the workers who brought suit. The first civil trial ended in a hung jury and mistrial after plaintiff Ed F. Kraus was charged with assault and battery in Salt Lake City. Kraus later was found innocent of criminal charges. During the second trial intoxicated company employees revealed to the plaintiff's attorney that Six Companies would be victorious because "they know how to fix juries." The judge refused to call for a new trial, but forty-eight additional suits sought $4.8 million in damages. The company decided to defuse the bombshell and settled out of court in January 1936 under undisclosed terms.[33]

Henry Kaiser's concern was for the corporate image rather than for working-class health, safety, and economic security. He complained to Secretary of the Interior Ray Lyman Wilbur about unfavorable publicity in the labor press. Six Companies had lost money, he claimed, as a result of work stoppages and additional services to workers, such as schools for their children subsidized from company coffers. The temporary company school was established in two vacant houses and an abandoned railroad shack for 800 students.[34]

In August 1932 Six Companies again tried to reduce wages.[35] Testifying before a House investigating committee on labor practices, Kaiser defended the wage rate paid by Six Companies. He described as impossibly confusing the Davis-Bacon law enacted by executive order in January 1932, which required a contractor to pay the "prevailing rate of wage" in a given locale. Few contractors, Kaiser said, would take on large contracts if they could then be fined, like Six Companies, for failing to comply with the law. He claimed that the four-dollars-a-day minimum wage paid at Boulder surpassed any other in the area. "The wage scale is probably satisfactory as far as Mr. Kaiser is concerned, but as far as organized labor is concerned it is not," the AFL representative retorted. "Now I venture to say that if you [Kaiser] had to work at Boulder Dam for $4 per day, you would not last fifteen minutes. You would have to go to a hospital."[36]

To reestablish peaceful relations with labor the company emphasized benefits beyond wages. By late summer of 1932 the planned community of Boulder City included eight dormitories, each for 172 men, more than 600 cottages, mess and recreation halls, a company store and offices, and a twenty-bed hospital. Living conditions and health care improved dramatically. No more fatalities occurred from dehydration.[37]

Company-sponsored reports pointed to the constant attention given to health and safety through a special department. In order to fulfill its workers' compensation obligations, the company operated Boulder City Hospital and several fully equipped first-aid stations, staffed by nurses around the clock. About a hundred passenger cars transported minor injury cases to the hospital and stations, with two Ford ambulances available for more serious ones. The press touted the medical facilities at the construction camp in the words of its "huge," "smiling" chief of staff, Dr. Wales A. Haas, as "the best equipped small hospital in the country." Five doctors and five nurses mostly treated fractures and cared also for workers' families. Unfortunately, the chief company physician did not last through completion of the dam. Board minutes recorded a resolution in March 1933 to select a new doctor for Boulder City "to replace the late Dr. Haas."[38]

Under California's workers' compensation laws, Garfield had to transfer injured workers almost 200 miles from Desert Center and the aqueduct to a Los Angeles hospital. He knew that only those who were not in critical condition could make the grueling trip. Starting with $2,500 in savings, he went into debt to build his own twelve-bed hospital. Even though the project would last only four years, he installed expensive venetian blinds and a complete air conditioning system, innovative for the time and place, to protect patients against the scorching climate. Radios, "decent" reading materials, and "attractive" nurses were other curative benefits Garfield described in his first hospital.[39]

Garfield's financial status meant that he was able to afford only himself, one nurse, a laundress, and a cook, and often did some of the work of the other three members of the staff. No additional income accumulated. The men were resentful and unable to pay medical expenses beyond that paid by workers' compensation insurance. At first Garfield did not even collect adequate workers' compensation fees because the industrial insurance companies objected to every claim and preferred to send the men to Los Angeles for treatment of serious (that is, lucrative) injuries. Debts mounted, and at one point his staff was not paid for seven months. A close colleague claims that Garfield used a rifle to chase a repossessor away from the station wagon that he used as an ambulance.[40]

Dr. Garfield's competence and dedication evident in the small desert hospital spurred creative assistance by Harold Hatch and Alonzo B. Ordway, officers of Industrial Indemnity Exchange, Garfield's first contacts with Six Companies and the Kaiser organization.[41] Hatch was an overseer of the industrial medical insurance held by Kaiser, the Six Companies, and others of the fifteen companies working on construction of the Colorado River reclamation projects at the Hoover Dam, Parker Dam, and Colorado River Aqueduct.[42] Since Garfield was losing money yet providing needed services and model facilities, Hatch proposed that Industrial Indemnity prepay to Garfield 17.5 percent of premiums, or $1.50 per worker per month, to treat industrial injuries. Hatch, Ordway, and Garfield conceived a plan for workers to pay dues of five cents a day in advance to cover illness and injury not related to work.[43]

A practical man, Garfield was not much concerned about the controversy brewing between Ross-Loos and the local medical society in his own hometown, nor did he give much thought to existing health plans. "I didn't know about 'em," he told an interviewer, and "wasn't particularly interested." He had heard about Ross-Loos in Los Angeles, and his uninformed opinion reflected the poor press given the county medical society affiliate of the AMA. Garfield pointed out that the "doctors didn't really like [Ross-Loos]," and that he himself "thought something was wrong with them." Garfield gave Ordway credit for suggesting prepayment for industrial medical care and recollected that in the early and mid-1930s he never thought much about Kaiser.[44]

In 1933 and 1934 Garfield struggled to make the paycheck deduction system work so that the supplement to workers' compensation would enable him to keep his medical operation afloat on the aqueduct. Five cents a day from 5,000 workers was enough to solve Garfield's financial problems. In the first few months only 500 men from one company made the voluntary contribution; others resisted until they got hurt and had to pay extra for care. The men earned from $0.45 to $1.10 an hour and had trouble budgeting enough for emergencies. Apparently impressed with Garfield's "beautiful little hospital," the employers came to his rescue. By the end of 1933 men from fourteen of the fifteen companies involved in some aspect of the project, including Kaiser and his partners of Six Companies headquartered at Hoover Dam, were paying their nickel a day. These funds were in addition to the flat rate the young doctor had negotiated with Industrial Indemnity from workers' compensation funds. Once he was out of the financial morass, Garfield added group practice to prepayment. These two practices, along with the new facilities he could build, he conceived as the basis of "*limitless* medical care"—the best available without the consideration of a fee for each service rendered.[45]

Garfield's only connection with Kaiser on the Colorado River project was through Industrial Indemnity. Kaiser himself was not involved with the day-to-day operation of the insurance consortium, nor was he mentioned in the Six Companies minutes as part of an executive committee to resolve financial contract difficulties over the agreement Garfield made with the partnership.[46]

Sixty percent of Garfield's income came from payroll deduction, 40 percent from workers' compensation. He paid off the $30,000 it had cost to build his first small hospital and built a second hospital in the Coachella Valley desert near Parker

Dam, and a third in 1935 at the Imperial Dam near Yuma, Arizona. Almost 100 percent of the workmen joined, and he employed ten physicians full time. Garfield paid off all equipment, all three hospitals, and the salaries of physicians and supporting staff, and ended his aqueduct enterprise with a reserve of $150,000. He returned to Los Angeles for further study with his mentors at the Los Angeles County Hospital, supplemented by a part-time teaching post at the University of Southern California. His intention was to enter private practice.[47] He appeared to be a traditionalist who, like other fledgling young doctors, had done a turn at contract practice merely to get a start during hard times. On the desert Garfield had not yet felt the chill of disapproval he would experience from independent physicians in urban areas of the Pacific Coast.

On 30 September 1935 President Roosevelt and the governors of six states journeyed to Boulder Dam, as the Roosevelt administration renamed Hoover Dam, for an official dedication ceremony. Henry J. Kaiser did not attend. He never again visited the immense structure that was the base of his subsequent success. Within a year he and the Six Companies partners were bidding on other big federal dam projects. Kaiser did not seem uniquely concerned about the welfare of his workers in the early and mid-1930s, nor particularly cognizant of the emergence of a new power alignment in industrial society in which organized labor played an integral role.

By the late 1930s, with a second federal project at Grand Coulee Dam, Kaiser company directors seemed to recognize that they stood at the vanguard of radical power shifts in labor-capital relations. In 1938 the magnate's son, Edgar Kaiser, asked Garfield to create a prepaid group medical program for 5,000 workers at Grand Coulee Dam. As Garfield prepared to leave Desert Center, workers on the project began to organize around militant union locals that formed the CIO in 1935.[48]

Militant unionism was the tie between the Kaiser industrial plans of the depression and war years, and the public plan offered on the West Coast in the postwar period. Like the WFM of an earlier era, organizing Pacific longshoremen were characteristic of the continuing aggressiveness of the western labor movement. The International Longshoremens' and Warehousemens' Union, formed in 1937, shut down the San Francisco waterfront twice in the 1930s. The longshoremen represented the brawny working-class community with which Kaiser identified.

Between 1919 and 1923 the IWW had enrolled hundreds of longshoremen in the revolutionary Maritime Transport Workers Industrial Union (MTW) and incited thousands more to strikes and work stoppages. A recent study attributes the radicalism and solidarity of Pacific maritime workers to their occupational recruitment from the highly mobile yet close-knit society of former lumbermen and seamen along the coast from Seattle, Washington, to San Pedro, California.[49] Newly forming union groups in the natural resource and maritime industries of the West replaced the lost ties to traditional community. Then in 1934 Harry Bridges of the International Longshoremen's Association led a general strike by 125,000 dockworkers on the San Francisco waterfront that shut down the premier port city for eighty-three days. It ended in bloodshed with two longshoremen dead and more than a hundred injured. The banner year of U.S. unionism was 1935, marked by passage of the Wagner Labor Relations and Social Security acts, and establishment of the CIO by John L. Lewis. Labor unionists in the resource industries were forceful in their continuing demands for occupational health and safety benefits. In 1937 and 1938, after another series of strikes and job actions, Bridges led the formation of the ILWU.[50]

The focus of federal efforts to harness the power of the western rivers shifted from the Colorado River to the Columbia, more than 600 miles to the north. Kaiser bid on the Bonneville project 40 miles east of Portland, and Grand Coulee, nestled in the dry transmountain region of the Cascades in Washington state, as Hoover Dam neared completion.[51] Kaiser got the construction job at Bonneville in 1934. At Grand Coulee the underwater construction, or lower dam, was awarded to Mason-Walsh-Atkinson and Kier (MWAK). The Henry J. Kaiser Company sponsored and managed a group known as Consolidated Builders, Inc., and won the second part of the contract in February 1938, for the superstructure known as the upper dam, along with its power houses and pumping plants.[52] Garfield moved his southern California desert experiment to Grand Coulee Dam where it became part of company legend.

The new Kaiser company took over from MWAK in 1938. Meanwhile a jerry-built and chaotic boomtown community, much like that near Las Vegas at Hoover Dam, sprang up in the vicinity of the Grand Coulee project. Journalists described scenes reminiscent of the Old West gold rush days. Refugees from the midwestern dust bowls and from poverty in all parts of the country came in "dilapidated automobiles" with "cart-like trailers" filled with worn household belongings and children. One engineer noted that "the functions of organized society lagged far behind the requirements which arose for them." By early 1936 the population of the hitherto isolated area was variously estimated at figures ranging from 9,000 to 12,000.[53]

A new town was formed as an amalgam of three older small communities—Grand Coulee City. Two new communities housed project employees. Coulee Dam was the government town for Bureau of Reclamation employees. Mason City was the construction town, built by stipulation in the government contract with MWAK and then with Consolidated Builders, for the contractor's crew and their families. The government camp housed only 525 residents. The contractor's town housed about 2,500 employees, with 1,500 in the men's dormitories and tents and 1,000 in separate houses, the hospital, hotel, and women's dormitories. Twelve hundred men were housed in twelve- and eight-room cabins with one toilet and shower, two men sleeping in each room. Each group of cabins also had access to a bathhouse. At the peak of 1936 construction MWAK employed 2,681 workers; since the total Mason City population, exclusive of tent residents, was only 2,100, almost 600 workers must have lived in the tents, been able to find lodging in the "free city" of Grand Coulee, or lived in what one writer called a "Hidden City" of the indigent and homeless. Mason City also had an exclusive "residence section" that housed executives such as Edgar Kaiser and his management partners. During construction the Bureau of

Reclamation acted in a supervisory capacity; afterward the dam was operated by government employees who remained there.[54] Thus, Coulee Dam was built as a permanent community; Mason City was temporary. The contrast illustrated a two-class community structure that prevailed for the project's duration.

Workers complained about poor conditions. Their irritation against historic abuses by owners at remote job sites and corporate-dominated construction towns began to have an impact. New Deal legislation, section 7a of the National Industrial Recovery Act and the Wagner Act of 1935, provided for public protection of the right to organize and for arbitration of disputes through the National Labor Relations Board (NLRB). The push for industrial unionism led by John L. Lewis and the CIO was evident at the Colorado River Aqueduct and at Grand Coulee Dam. Kaiser executives saw the need to respond to this newly organized force and began to view the isolated worker communities from an enlightened perspective.

Partnership with government was a double-edged sword. The western companies that built Hoover, Grand Coulee, and the other massive reclamation projects of the 1930s were launched with the New Deal.[55] At the same time that federal projects boosted corporate expansion, however, they acted as a strong regulatory force. Kaiser could not afford to flout federal regulation of the terms and conditions of labor. The Hoover Dam project represented an initial period of recalcitrance evident in Kaiser's 1935 testimony before Congress in opposition to the Davis-Bacon Act, and in the battle waged by company police against union radicals. A more positive capital-labor relationship developed at Grand Coulee Dam.

As Harry Bridges's longshoremen shut down the San Francisco waterfront for the second time in five years, the economy again dipped, and 1937 was a turbulent year in national labor relations. A threatened strike at Grand Coulee Dam in August 1937 was averted, yet agitation by the newly organized CIO United Dam Construction Workers Local 295 continued against Kaiser's predecessors for violation of Public Works Administration (PWA) and minimum wage regulations, and for its closed-shop agreement with the AFL affiliates. Edgar Kaiser arrived in March 1938 to take over construction from MWAK amid deplorable housing conditions and pent-up worker resentment. Much farther south 600 strikers of CIO affiliate Aqueduct, Subway, and Tunnel Workers' Local 270, perhaps threatened by the loss of jobs as the Colorado River project ended, blocked the road between Parker Dam and Desert Center, where Sidney Garfield had built his first hospital.[56]

Workers fought minimum wage violations under Davis-Bacon, but medical care was an issue as well. The original Washington State workers' compensation law of 1911 did not require the employer to provide medical care, but a 1917 amendment required employer and employee to share equally the cost for care of industrial accidents and injury. In Washington and Oregon employers could contract with physicians for a flat fee for industrial injuries rather than making payments to a state fund. As it had on the Hoover Dam and Colorado River Aqueduct projects, the Kaiser company chose this option at Grand Coulee Dam. It was difficult for companies to attract doctors to isolated areas, and employers often allowed physicians to extend medical care programs beyond treatment for industrial injuries to comprehensive care. Employees paid for this through the same wage check-off system as on the aqueduct project in southern California. In Washington employees paid half the cost of industrial accident cases and the total cost of other services, including care of dependents.[57]

The unions at Grand Coulee still were disgruntled over the state of affairs under Kaiser's predecessors. They harbored the historic bias against corporate medicine and the company doctor and did not want the Kaiser company to operate the Mason City Hospital. When Edgar Kaiser arrived to head the project management team in March 1938, he persuaded union members to give the company a chance to improve conditions. On the advice of Harold Hatch and Alonzo Ordway of Industrial Indemnity, he had Ordway contact Sidney Garfield. Both Kaiser and Garfield were dubious of the other's good reputation. Anxious to get into private practice in Los

Angeles, Garfield insisted to Ordway that he was not interested in a contract at the dam. Finally, as a "favor," he traveled to Portland to meet Edgar Kaiser, who convinced him to drive up to Spokane and the Grand Coulee as a short-term consultant.

The drive took several hours. "By the time we got there," Garfield admitted, "I had lost all my antipathy . . . and wanted to help him." He saw many advantages to the Grand Coulee proposal. In contrast to the situation on the Colorado River Aqueduct, where he had cared for between 5,000 and 7,000 men strung out over 200 miles, at Grand Coulee the worker population was "all in one spot with a contemporary community built up all around them." Here was a place to experiment with Garfield's ideal of a prepaid group practice. He might thus pick up where he had left off in the Southwest desert.[58]

Edgar Kaiser's congeniality and his view of the community at the dam site dissolved Garfield's doubts. But Kaiser remained unconvinced of Garfield's potential. For one thing he was startled by Sidney Garfield's physical appearance. Ordway's son later described him as a "loudly dressed southern California type." Garfield was a misfit in the drab depression era. He later told an interviewer that he did not recall what he wore, only that he did not wear black; and he did have rather "shocking" red hair. Edgar called Ordway after his first glimpse, to tell him that Garfield did not look like a physician. Ordway encouraged him to refrain from judgment until he got to know the doctor better.[59]

A small eighty-five-bed hospital already existed at the Grand Coulee Dam site, built by the contractors during the first phase of construction. But the medical care arrangement between the company and half a dozen physicians was highly unsatisfactory to the unions. Like the construction of the government and company employee towns, medical care was based on a two-class structure. Workers had a health plan paid for by wage deductions and workers' compensation, but they felt that the doctors lavished most attention on the private practice by which they supplemented their company salaries. De Kruif writes that union members claimed they were "like dirt under the doctors' feet."[60]

When Garfield arrived at the Mason City Hospital he found numerous cases of unimproved chronic infections. Injured workers had to make their way to the second floor for treatment, in poorly designed outpatient facilities. Surgery was conducted in open areas where patients in dirty work clothes wandered in and out. Anxious to rectify the situation and create a prepaid, multispecialty group medical program in the "stable" but turbulent community, Garfield considered it "a tremendous opportunity" to expand his desert experiment. He agreed to a contract with Consolidated Builders as Sidney R. Garfield and Associates, a sole proprietorship, to provide medical service at Mason City Hospital.

Garfield's first problem was putting together his group of physicians. The medical program at Grand Coulee did not have a good reputation, and Washington physicians would not leave established practices for an uncertain and temporary contract with Garfield, even for $500 to $600 a month at a time when many doctors were averaging only $3,000 net annual income. Furthermore, the doctors under contract had no overhead or staff to pay, and they got housing, food, and bonuses if the project was profitable, benefits far greater than young physicians could expect to earn in private practice with its substantial start-up costs.

Kaiser publicists write that Garfield "barnstormed the country," wiring and telephoning long-distance in the Kaiser "grand manner." He "flew from coast to coast," and within six months he was able to create what he called a "little Mayo Clinic."[61] Those actually involved with recruitment tell of a less dramatic, more geographically circumscribed process. There were only seven medical program doctors for nearly 10,000 workers and family members. Five were Californians: Garfield recruited a fellow resident, Dr. Wallace Neighbor, from the Los Angeles County Hospital, then persuaded three young physicians who had just completed residencies at Stanford to join him—Cecil Cutting as chief of surgery, another surgeon, and an obstetrician/gynecologist. The other two physicians were general practitioners, one from Michigan and Dr. Eugene Wiley of Iowa, Garfield's fellow medical student at the University of Iowa.

While Garfield collected his group of physicians, he supervised the rebuilding of the Mason City Hospital with three modern operating rooms and air-conditioning. He insisted on these improvements even though they cost the Kaisers and their associates $100,000, okaying the expensive cooling system without company approval. Edgar Kaiser agreed to pay for it after the fact, but he warned the doctor not to take such financial initiative again, a retreat from earlier assurances that the patients' welfare was a priceless commodity.[62]

How did the working-class patients fit into Garfield's new medical community? Henry Kaiser, an ambivalent witness to union organizing at Hoover Dam in the early part of the decade, now committed himself to establishing good labor relations. Garfield later remembered that at Grand Coulee Kaiser "surprised" him with his views on the role of unions in the new industrial order. "It was his feeling," Garfield said, "that unions were absolutely necessary in the industrial world of today. He felt that the unions were a great contribution to that; he felt they were necessary and he was 100 percent for them."[63]

Upon the Kaiser team's arrival at Mason City, Garfield set up a prepaid voluntary health plan whereby the men had fifty cents a week deducted from their paychecks for nonwork-related care, about seven cents a day. Added to the percentage of workers' compensation premium prepaid by the insurance company, the workers' prepayment covered virtually unlimited medical care. Garfield reported that the unions were won over quickly and "were so happy with the services we rendered that they took over the job of marketing it to the workers themselves. We didn't have to raise a finger; [union officers] would sign them all up."[64]

Yet there were drawbacks to the company-administered welfare system. The seven cents a day for health care was only one company levy on the workers. A sample payroll record shows that a skilled worker earning $60 a week gross pay in the early summer of 1938 had 45 cents deducted from the total for "hospital dues." This deduction was relatively minor in relation to several others: federal and state social and health care security, 80 cents a week; house rent, $8.75; electricity,

$4.80; "stores," $15.82; and "miscellaneous," $2.50. These charges left only a little more than one-third of the worker's weekly income intact and explains labor's negative perception of the company town. Through the payment and provision system at self-contained, isolated job sites, the company kept a firm hand on every aspect of working-class life and leisure.[65]

Union leaders encouraged participation in the health plan but recognized the dichotomy in service. Though care for the approximately five thousand workers improved, a substantial front-door, nonplan patient practice still boosted doctor and hospital income. De Kruif is frank about the enormous benefits to Garfield and Associates of the traditional fee-for-service practice for workers' dependents, the government supervisors who lived at Coulee Dam, and the merchants and others who provided concessions to the community. The latter included those Cutting called "whore house" and "gunshop" entrepreneurs.[66]

As Sidney Garfield put "plenty of money on the books," worker resentment rose. Family care was the subject of rising benefit demands through the remainder of the twentieth century. Workers now received adequate medical care, but their families did not. There was no county or charity hospital, and families were involuntarily dependent on the care set up by the company at Mason City. The workers rarely saved enough from paychecks for such unanticipated events as family illness and injury. According to de Kruif, the doctors were the villains in these instances. "Dr. Jekylls and Mr. Hydes," they were admired for their prepaid services to the workers and vilified as "gold diggers" for the "exorbitant" fees charged wives and children. Garfield described the dilemma this created for everyone: "We had to take care of them [the families]. We had to bill them for the services, and they just didn't have the money to pay for it."[67]

Although Cutting and Garfield recalled the problems less dramatically than did de Kruif, they both emphasized that all groups concerned—the unions, the doctors, and Edgar Kaiser himself—saw the advantage of including families in prepayment. Garfield declared that the unions forced the move toward a family plan by again threatening to strike unless one was instituted. Edgar Kaiser later was proud that his workers never actually went out on strike. Family medical care was the first trial of his ability to work out a cooperative agreement, and he prompted Garfield to help him design a way to provide such services. The concept was untried. No families had been involved on the desert job, and Grand Coulee was the first time the Kaisers themselves were completely responsible for worker medical care. The two men initially "picked figures out of the air" in deciding cost. They tried fifty cents a week for wives and twenty-five cents for each child as subscription fees to be added to the payroll deduction for the men.[68]

According to de Kruif, for over three months after the unions announced the "family plan," it was an "unexpected flop." Only 10 to 15 percent of the families enrolled while most waited until they were actually sick to sign up. Obviously the insurance principles of spreading risk and payment through an average population would not work if the only plan members were sick people. After union leaders became more actively involved, an estimated 90 percent of the families joined, leaving only government employees and inhabitants of the "Hidden City" without coverage.[69]

As the plan became highly regarded in the community, the end result was more business and a higher income for the doctors through the front-door practice among nonplan residents in the surrounding area. Perhaps 10,000 people employed by the government or who had established shops and services around the project site did not belong to the plan, in addition to 5,000 workers and their dependents who did. That Garfield's program offered the only available medical care in the vicinity and that its reputation was good meant that it was used by many private patients. One report credits this private fee-for-service complement with a 10 percent rise in doctor and hospital income in the first two years of the service.[70]

At the Mason City Hospital leading medical program administrators were brought together into a working relationship, and the basic principles of Kaiser program development established. Most important, Henry J. Kaiser became personally acquainted with Garfield, his colleagues, and their ideas.

Henry Kaiser was only a fleeting observer of the medical program at Grand Coulee, but Garfield recollected one visit to the dam site in 1938 when he met with "the boss." After spending practically an entire day touring the facilities and talking with the staff, Kaiser made a proclamation that astounded Garfield. He announced that if the plan was "half as good" as Garfield said it was "it should be made available to everybody in the whole country." Garfield was shocked by the thought of such a monumental and seemingly impossible undertaking. He had just "gone through so much hell" setting up the "little place" at Grand Coulee. How could he be expected to "take care of the whole country?" Kaiser reassured the young doctor that he would have "plenty of help" and would be expected only to set an example, establish a model for others to emulate, not do it all himself.[71]

Dr. Cutting recalled that Garfield was only at Mason City about every fourth weekend during the four-year project at Grand Coulee, while Cutting had only every sixth weekend off duty. According to another observer, Garfield remained busy back in Los Angeles working on a number of nonmedical side enterprises, such as a Buick agency and a string of apartment buildings, in addition to keeping his hand in professional practice. Garfield thought he would be returning to his hometown in southern California when the dam project ended.[72]

The most stunning corporate accomplishment at Grand Coulee Dam was technological rather than humanitarian. On 22 March 1941, the Nez Perce chief pulled the switch at the west powerhouse and sent 20,000 kilowatts of power over the transmission lines to the Nespeelem Indian Reservation. Consolidated Builders hastily dismantled its operations at the dam, including the Mason City Hospital and the health plan. Many of the construction personnel had left the area, and Kaiser management asked "to be relieved of the responsibility of operating the town" by 1 November. The contractors wanted to transfer the hospital personnel to the new Kaiser shipbuilding plant at Vancouver, Washington. In a telegram to the Bureau of Reclamation (BOR), the supervising engineer stressed the need to execute a new contract for running the hospital because the current personnel were "unwilling to delay further Vancouver assignments." The BOR agreed in the original contract to take over all of Mason City when the dam was complete for $25,000. The bureau now had to contract with other doctors to take over the hospital.

Under the Mason City Hospital Corporation, organized as a subsidiary of Consolidated Builders by Garfield, Cutting, and their colleagues, the health plan was operated at "a very substantial profit." Supervising engineer W. A. Banks reported that the combined incomes from subcontracts with the State Department of Labor and Industry, and contracts negotiated with individual workers for fifty cents a week through the AFL unions, produced a profit in 1941 of about $24,000. Government officials found the contractor's accounting system complex in its division between hospitalization and "medical care," its tax shelters, and the way it turned its workers' compensation obligations to advantage.[73]

BOR supervisors were impressed with the contractor's speed and "diligence" in completing the dam project as the country geared for war. The newly formed voluntary Northwest National Defense Council, whose organizing convention was held in Mason City in July 1940, expressed "its deepest appreciation for the cooperation and support" of Consolidated Builders in the speedy completion of the dam, vital to the regional defense effort.[74] The Kaiser team thus left for the Pacific Coast with the support of the local community and with the aura of patriotic endeavor that carried it through the war years.

The enormous scale of the reclamation projects added to the Bunyanesque image of Henry Kaiser and the visibility of his industrial communities and cast Kaiser's work force in bold relief. Just as the railroads joined the rugged and transient industrial populations of the West in the second half of the nineteenth century, water was the natural connecting force for the spreading network of industrial workers in the desert and maritime West. The huge Kaiser reclamation projects carried this hardy population into the mushrooming port cities of Portland, Vancouver, and San Francisco. In southern California they fanned out from the steel plant at Fontana in San Bernardino County westward to Los Angeles.

But the Kaiser team moved under twin storm clouds. One

portended professional antagonism against government intervention in national health care and the other, world war. Contemporary AMA rhetoric combined images of the two. The association also opposed group practice and medical cooperatives as "nothing more than contract practice arrangements which violate the principles of medical ethics."[75] On the same grounds it opposed any form of compulsory state insurance, which during the depression had seemed certain of passage. Chief AMA editor Morris Fishbein reduced the issues to their ideological essentials. "We object to compulsory sickness insurance," he wrote in the *New England Journal of Medicine* in March 1939, as Hitler marched through Eastern Europe,

not only because it degrades the quality of medical service, not only because it enslaves the medical profession of the country . . . but because primarily it is the first insidious approach to the breakdown of the democratic system of government. Give anybody the right to interfere thus intimately with the lives of the people, to pay for them the physician, whether or not the physician is selected by the patient, and you have the first step toward totalitarianism, whether it be under the name of Fascism, or Communism.[76]

In 1939 Kaiser began his big shipbuilding contracts on the West Coast, headquartered in Oakland on the east side of San Francisco Bay. By 1940 union membership in the San Francisco Bay Area was 27 percent of the labor force when it was only 17 percent nationwide. Meanwhile, only 9 percent (twelve million) of the population had any kind of hospital insurance and only 5 percent (seven million) had medical service coverage, with more than half for surgical. Professional demographics and income remained unfavorable in San Francisco, a barometer of practitioners' status in the region.[77] A multitude of demographic, economic, and political factors converging at the Kaiser shipyards on the West Coast would change the regional shape of U.S. medicine and health.

2 Shipyard Communities and Occupational Health

Four Kaiser shipyards and a prefabrication plant have been built on the waterfront. One hundred thousand people live where 24,000 lived before. Huge barrackslike public-housing projects cover the mud flats between the harbor and the town. . . . The truth [about Richmond, California] was plain in the crowded schools, operating in three and sometimes four shifts; in the filthy trailer camps around the edges of town; in the untended children swarming the muddy compounds of the housing projects; and in the puzzled faces of uprooted, unwelcomed Oklahomans and Texans.

—Katherine Hamill, "Richmond Took a Beating"

KAISER INDUSTRIES MOVED FROM THE TINY, remote "urban oases" of the dam projects to the new Kaiser shipyards on the teeming urban Pacific Coast.[1] As the industrialist transformed the landscape along the northeastern shore of San Francisco Bay from Richmond to Oakland, during World War II the Kaiser industrial health plan transformed the regional structure of medical care. Despite the obstacles of enormous population growth, social turmoil, and the antagonism of the local

medical establishment, Kaiser's Dr. Sidney Garfield established a health plan to serve nearly 200,000 shipworkers on a
scale forty times that of the earlier Kaiser dam projects.

Between 1940 and 1947 the population of the three West
Coast states increased 30 percent faster than the national aver-
age. From 1940 to 1950 California increased 35 percent;
Washington, 27 percent; and Oregon, 29 percent. Five of the
nation's ten "congested population areas," designated by the
federal government for special attention, were on the West
Coast: San Diego, Los Angeles, San Francisco, Portland, and
Seattle. Kaiser's Liberty ship contracts with the U.S. Maritime
Commission (USMC) stimulated the population explosions in
the San Francisco and Portland areas. Oakland, the location of
Kaiser corporate headquarters, grew by 20 percent. Richmond was a small town of under 24,000 twelve miles north,
also in the East San Francisco Bay Area. The location of four
Kaiser shipyards, it grew by more than 100,000 inhabitants
from 1940 to 1944. Workers migrated to the two San Francisco Bay cities mainly from the South and Midwest: 19 percent from Texas, Oklahoma, Arkansas, and Louisiana; 14
percent from Michigan, Illinois, Indiana, and Ohio. Local and
federal housing agencies constructed thousands of living units
on the flatlands along the bay, creating "shipyard ghettos,"
according to one analyst, that entrenched ethnic, racial, and
socioeconomic segregation of new from old residents. The
multiethnic working-class population that evolved during the
war settled near the rail lines and docks, as middle-class whites
clustered in the eastern hillside areas.[2]

The Kaiser plan linked industrial and public health medicine, a dual concept to which early Kaiser plan physicians were
committed. Two of Garfield's first recruits to the shipyards'
health team in 1942 were Morris F. Collen and Cecil C. Cutting. Formerly at Grand Coulee, Cutting now was Garfield's
chief of staff in northern California. He did every type of
surgery, including mammary artery implants in cardiology,
and was chief surgeon in orthopedics and neurosurgery. Collen
focused on the infectious lung diseases (he himself was eliminated from military service as a result of bronchial asthma and
allergies) historically prevalent among the working poor of

the textile and mining industries. He devoted his career to clinical research experiments and to the care of patients with pneumonia and tuberculosis. He was the linchpin of postwar Permanente programs in the medical research field, and later in multiphasic screening of the longshoremen. He later defined the field of computer medicine, used in multiphasic screening of ILWU members, as a public health technology.[3]

From 1942 to 1944 the shipyard physicians were swamped with trauma cases and a huge acute care patient load. They chose to remain in occupational group practice as specialization segmented the profession with rapid scientific advances, new specialty board approval procedures, and a labyrinth of elite educational requirements. U.S. hospital patients were increasingly affluent in the 1940s, and hospitals focused on "knowledge-based" services requiring technological sophistication, rather than on providing broad access to care.[4]

During the war Permanente general practitioners were still in the mainstream of their profession, with 76.5 percent reporting themselves as general practitioners or part-time specialists; two decades later over half of U.S. doctors declared specialties.[5] Cutting and Collen bridged the gap that widened dramatically in the 1940s and 1950s between general practice and specialization. The public health and group consciousness of Permanente leaders at the Kaiser shipyards set them apart from most U.S. doctors and were critical elements in developing a group identity and medical culture that differed from that of the majority of U.S. physicians who remained in solo fee-for-service practice.

After Hitler's invasion of Poland in September 1939, Kaiser went into partnership with Todd Shipyards Corporation to build five C-1 cargo ships under contract with the U.S. Maritime Commission. The British government signed a contract with the Todd-Kaiser partnership at the end of 1940 to build thirty ships at its Richmond yard in the East San Francisco Bay Area. In January 1941 Admiral Howard L. Vickery initiated the Liberty ship program. Early the same month newspapers announced that Kaiser had acquired eighty-seven acres as the location for the Oregon Shipbuilding Corporation plant. The first four Liberty keels were laid at Richmond in April 1941; on 16 August Hull Number One, the *Ocean Vanguard*, slipped down the Kaiser-built shipways.[6]

A month before the Japanese attacked Pearl Harbor on 7 December 1941, Kaiser formed the Permanente Metals Corporation, bought out the Todd interests, and became sole owner at Richmond and of Oregon Shipbuilding Corporation in Portland. In 1943 Kaiser added three more yards: Richmond Number Four, and in the Portland-Vancouver area, Swan Island and Kaiser-Vancouver. To bolster the precarious steel supply for the ships, Kaiser established a steel mill at Fontana. The Kaiser yards produced more than a quarter of all USMC ships built between 1941 and 1945, 1,460 ships, in addition to the thirty for Britain.[7] From Fontana, Richmond, and Portland-Vancouver, the Kaiser medical program burgeoned during the war and into the postwar era.

Although the shipyard communities at Richmond and Portland-Vancouver were constructed as parts of existing cities, Richmond was so altered by the national defense industries as to become unrecognizable within two years, from 1941 to 1943. It had been founded in the late 1890s as the outlet to San Francisco Bay for the Santa Fe transcontinental rail line, and the site of the Standard Oil refinery at the end of the pipeline from Bakersfield. In the 1930s development of Richmond's natural port drew Ford Motor Company, and tank storage for the Richfield Oil Corporation, a cannery, and other food industries.

In June 1941 new defense industry workers in the Bay Area numbered 101,000; in June 1942, 171,000. By April 1943 growth was dispersed into all the East and North Bay counties of San Francisco, San Mateo, Alameda, Contra Costa, and Marin, with a total migration of 269,000 people to the manufacturing industries. Most of the 221,600 new workers entered shipbuilding, with almost half in Richmond. The Richmond population rose from 23,642 in 1940 to 130,000 by April 1943, growing to more than 8.6 times the small size it had maintained for almost half a century. Portland's population jumped from 160,000 to 359,000 with an additional 100,000 people arriving in outlying communities. As government fueled the critical shipbuilding industry with almost $4.8 billion in contracts, employment climbed to over 1.7 million shipyard workers nationwide at the wartime peak in 1943; about 12 percent were employed by the Kaiser companies.[8]

Housing and urban services at Richmond were woefully inadequate from 1941 through the middle of 1942, when the Federal Public Housing Authority, the U.S. Maritime Commission, and the Kaiser companies began an intensive housing construction program. Workers were encouraged to come to the area without their families. Over 550,000 names appeared in the Kaiser Richmond personnel files alone, as labor turnover and workers' dependents swelled the transient working-class population to enormous proportions.[9]

Kaiser management sought the easiest route in relations with the newly empowered union movement. In April 1941 the AFL Metal Trades Council negotiated the West Coast Master's Agreement with Kaiser, guaranteeing an AFL closed shop in the shipyards after only a few hundred men were hired. The International Brotherhood of Boilermakers, Iron Ship Builders, Welders and Helpers of America thereafter controlled 65 percent of the jobs classified at the Kaiser yards. They were a strong counterweight to corporate authority but also enforced AFL discriminatory practices. By war's end, nearly all of the 90,000 Kaiser workers in the Northwest were represented by the AFL Metal Trades Council and forty-seven union locals. The dominant figure was Tom Ray of Portland Boilermaker's Local 72, described by *Fortune* magazine as "the largest, richest, and most glamorous union in the country."[10] Industry executives believed they had to keep peace with Local 72 for optimal productivity.

In January 1941 Henry Kaiser, Jr., telephoned Garfield in Los Angeles and asked him to set up a medical plan for the rapidly growing labor force in Richmond Yard One. The population explosion overwhelmed the twenty-nine local doctors. By June there were 16,000 new workers, and the town had nearly doubled in size. Garfield sought contracts with insurance companies approved by the USMC to carry the required workers' compensation insurance, as sole proprietor of a medical and hospital plan for industrial illness and injury. He financed it with 17.5 percent of the premium payment from the insurance carriers, supplemented by a prepayment plan for individual workers at a rate of fifty cents a week to cover nonindustrial medical needs. Garfield figured he could provide comprehensive care for less than 2 percent of the worker's annual wage for an individual and less than 4 percent for a family. Working-class families paid almost 4.5 percent of their income for minimal care based on traditional fee-for-service, private practice, and separate hospitalization.[11]

Despite an acute labor shortage that developed within six months after Pearl Harbor, the company more than doubled its work force to 30,000 by aggressive nationwide recruitment. Recruiters brought workers by railroad from every region of the nation. Within two years the Richmond Yard One payroll of 4,000 leaped to 93,000 in the four yards combined. By December 1943 employment at the Vancouver Yard peaked at 38,695. Oregon Shipbuilding and Swan Island added about 60,000 additional workers to the Kaiser force.[12]

Overcrowding caused great mental and physical stress for those in the mammoth working-class migration, manifest in the labor turnover, absenteeism, and general social unrest in the shipyards that were major problems both for employers and the war effort.[13] A skilled shipworker at Richmond who earned $61 a week spent $18.50 for food, $8.50 for rent, and $2.45 for transportation. But these wages could not buy adequate housing and services. New arrivals to the area had to set up tents or live in lofts in abandoned warehouses and in shacks built of scrap lumber. Sewage was piped into San Francisco Bay untreated and overflowed manholes, at times seeping into basements and streets.[14]

The housing crisis peaked at Portland-Vancouver in July 1942. Edgar Kaiser complained to the USMC that workers left because they could not find living space. Portland mayor Earl Riley let the young Kaiser choose replacements for the local housing authority while city planners grumbled at the location and quality of the housing construction projects. Thus bypassing local officials, Edgar contracted for construction of dormitories for 4,000 men, more than 10,000 one- to three-room "war apartments" for couples, and almost 9,000 single or duplex houses.[15] Planning for Vanport, called by the company "the largest war housing project in the world," began in September in an effort to integrate the sprawling employee housing network. The company town was known as Kaiserville until the local Housing Authority dubbed it Vanport, as the offspring of its two parent cities. By mid-July 1943 the population was 31,500 people. Bus transportation was provided for each of the three area shipyards. The Vancouver yard was less than a mile away, but Swan Island and Oregon Shipbuilding were almost six miles from the worker community.[16]

The shipyard press described Vanport as a 647-acre model community, built out of swampland on the banks of the Columbia River. New facilities enhanced the sense of community, called the "Vanport way of life."[17] Other accounts were far less laudatory. A congressional subcommittee reported that Vanport was "shoddily constructed." A former resident charged that built on an "inadequately filled swamp" between two major rivers, Vanport "was never more than a huge collection of crackerbox houses strung together fast and cheap."[18]

The company called Garfield back to Richmond from Los Angeles a second time in early 1942, as he prepared to embark with the Southern California Army Reserve Corps for India. He agreed to serve as a temporary medical consultant. Workers swamped local doctors' offices. Company officials told Garfield that the company had trouble getting injured workers into local hospitals, nor could they get appointments with private doctors. Even though he had only a month before he was due to embark for India, Garfield began to establish a medical plan at Richmond, as he had conceived it earlier. Kaiser officials submitted it to the insurance carriers as mandatory, with the full backing of management and labor.[19]

On 1 March 1942 offices opened at the Medical Center Building in Oakland. Industrial care was provided to 20,000 workers in Richmond Yards One and Three by six doctors and six nurses employed by Sidney R. Garfield and Associates. On 1 June the supplemental Permanente Health Plan opened at Richmond Yard One, with medical services provided under Garfield's sole proprietorship. Construction began on the Richmond Field Hospital with ten beds and an outpatient department subsidized by the Federal Works Administration (FWA) and run by Permanente on a rental agreement. Overflow patients went to Oakland under a temporary arrangement with Merritt Hospital. Garfield looked for an old hospital building to renovate as he had done at Mason City and commenced negotiations with Merritt for their Fabiola Hospital twelve miles from the yards. Merritt agreed to provide twenty beds at Merritt for Garfield's patients until renovation was complete.[20]

The main Fabiola building had burned down. The part that remained was a four-story concrete structure also partly demolished because the FWA had begun to convert it into a dormitory. The federal project was abandoned halfway through reconstruction. Garfield conducted a tour of the building with Henry Kaiser, fearing its condition would appall the industrialist. The two men started on the top floor and walked down because the elevators did not work. Kaiser was silent until they were at the bottom and asked Garfield, "What's the matter? Don't you think I have any imagination?" Garfield explained the sum he needed to Kaiser in a rushed one-hour meeting aboard the train from Oakland to Sacramento as Kaiser sped eastward to Washington, D.C. Although most bankers considered hospital construction loans poor credit risks, Kaiser had a banker as well known for risk taking in the financial world as Kaiser was in construction. Amadeo P. Giannini, founder and chair of the Bank of America, built his institution's stature on liberal lending and confidence in small innovative businesses. He agreed to support Garfield's hospital venture with a $250,000 loan backed by Kaiser.[21]

Kaiser used Washington connections to obtain Garfield's release from the army hospital unit he had signed up for with his friend Raymond Kay in southern California. Garfield recalled that "Ray was mad as hell at me" until he conceived of a way the separation from Garfield might eventually be beneficial to them both. He suggested that Garfield start a nonprofit health care foundation to create funds to start a health plan with him in Los Angeles after the war. This appealed to Garfield because his family and educational roots were there, and he made the commitment.[22]

Garfield took the idea to Kaiser, whom he met in Sacra-

mento on his return from Washington aboard the City of San
Francisco, now heading west. His attorney, also aboard, cau-
tioned that it could not be done. Always impatient with unpleasant advice, Kaiser snapped that he was "sick and tired of
having lawyers tell me things we can't do." He told Garfield,
"Now you tell me how we can do it. That's your job."[23]

As the housing crisis at both Portland-Vancouver and Richmond escalated, the Permanente Foundation was established
in July 1942, the name borrowed from the Spanish conquis-
tadors' name for the creek at the site of Kaiser's first cement
plant in California. Henry Kaiser gave the name to several
Kaiser enterprises at the wish of his first wife, Bess Fosburgh.
Kaiser trustees formed the Northern Permanente Foundation
the same year in Vancouver, Washington, to finance construction of a new hospital for workers at the Portland-Vancouver
shipyards. Southern Permanente was created for the Fontana
steel mill, designed to handle 3,500 employees and their families.

On 1 August 1942 the first Permanente Hospital opened in
Oakland with seventy beds, thirteen doctors, twenty-five
nurses, and thirty-two other employees. Within three weeks
the ten-bed Richmond Field Hospital also opened, with seventy-five beds added a month later. Yards One and Three
thus had a medical program for Kaiser employees by August
1942. Another health plan was opened in January 1943 at
Yard Four. Demand quickly exceeded program capacity.
Thousands of employees were covered only by regular
workers' compensation insurance while Permanente Health
Plan organizers worked frantically to add staff and facilities
sufficient to handle more members.[24]

The Oakland Permanente Hospital was filled immediately
beyond capacity. Garfield and Kaiser decided to enlarge it
only three months after Kaiser signed the $250,000 note. By
the end of the first year of operation Garfield reported to the
Permanente trustees that $500,000 of the $700,000 debt for
construction and equipment was paid. The industrialist demanded that the bankers themselves guarantee another loan
for $300,000.[25]

A month after the opening of Oakland Permanente Hospital and the creation of the Northwest's Northern Permanente

Foundation, the 10 September 1942 issue of the *Bo's'n's Whistle* announced the opening of the new 300-bed Northern Permanente Hospital located one mile east of the Vancouver shipyard. Garfield designed a central work space encircled by patient and operating rooms with peripheral corridors for visitors and for bringing in patients. Decorated in "soft grey-green colors," each two-bed room had toilet facilities and individual clothes closets; most rooms had a view of the Columbia River and the mountains. Eventually the Northern Permanente Foundation opened clinics at two area housing projects and employed 43 doctors and 190 nurses. Dr. Wallace Neighbor was medical director.[26]

Richmond conditions were deplorable throughout 1943. There was no shower, sewer, or trash collection system in places where many workers settled, so refuse was thrown out anywhere. Outdoor privies without roofs each served about one hundred people. Trailer parks where more than 2,000 people lived were put adjacent to dumps and swamps.[27] Henry Kaiser tried determinedly to keep a derogatory report on Richmond from appearing in *Fortune* magazine in February 1945. In frantic letters to the publishers he charged that the proposed article was biased and unpatriotic and would hurt the war effort by lowering the shipworkers' morale. Though the article appeared, with photographs by Ansel Adams of the new multiethnic Richmond population, the author relieved Kaiser management of blame for the squalor in which workers lived. She pointed out that "the Kaiser management has tried in many ways to provide satisfactory living conditions for the people it brought into Richmond" and that "the city government admits that Mr. Kaiser has been cooperative. The nursery schools near the yards are excellent, and so is the Permanente Field Hospital," although the Richmond School District administered the preschools, funded by the USMC.[28] Viewed through middle-class eyes conditions were less than desirable. From the perspective of many of the inhabitants, however, they were an improvement over depression-era living conditions in the South and Midwest. At least there was an attempt to instill community spirit.

Worker enrollment in the Permanente Health Plan was not

left to chance. Management bombarded workers with information and created a check-off system for dues collection that made membership almost automatic. Every employee received letters and pamphlets to explain the plan and sign-up procedures. A loudspeaker system and announcements in the shipyard press gave extra reminders.[29] Enrollment was a patriotic duty. Management humanized the rhetoric, but it reflected the powerful utilitarian determinant at the core of this merger of industrial medicine and public health. "Your health is your most priceless possession and this Plan is designed to help you keep it," management instructed the workforce.

Based on national experience, it is estimated that when the Richmond Shipyards are in full production, unless preventative measures are taken, a total of 720,000 working days a year will be lost due to accidents occurring away from work and due to illness. With those lost days, you could build ten ships. With those lost days, you could earn more than four million dollars. Such waste is tragic when the Nation is fighting for its very life and when ships are in greatest need. For the lack of even *one* ship to carry vital war materials to some desperate group of fighting men may well cost them their lives and rob them of their chance to win a splendid victory.[30]

The cost of fulfilling this national duty was only fifty to sixty cents a week per worker; that is, when enrollment in the Permanente Health Plan was available.

Kaiser addressed workers as equal participants in a cooperative and patriotic endeavor. In the 1930s, Socialist party member Algie Martin Simons, in collaboration with Dr. Nathan Sinai on a study of health care, expressed an orthodox theory of industrial medicine based on common precepts of economic efficiency, regarding the worker as a production unit: "Modern 'scientifically' managed industry, with its stop-watch standardized assembly lines, quick turnover, high overhead, and sharply specialized workers demands continuity of operation."[31] Kaiser implemented theories of industrial efficiency in a patriotic and humanistic guise. Managers sought to remedy low productivity, excess turnover, and absenteeism through health planning that included nutrition, child care, prepared meals for female workers, and voluntary participation in the

Permanente Health Plan. The organizing principles of competition and broad working-class access to preventive medicine and ambulatory care redefined the "sick role." What had been passivity and dependence became mutual responsibility for individual health and safety.[32] Kaiser cajoled workers with sticks as well as carrots for improved productivity. The company conducted studies to identify "malingerers" and "gold bricks" in their excessive use of the first-aid stations and medical facilities. The patient should have an active desire to return to the production line. The physician was likewise transformed from a patriarchal healer with mystical powers to a facilitator in the maintenance of health.

Garfield had difficulty keeping up with demand because of the large and rapid population growth in the region coupled with facility and staff shortages. He had to combine several different programs to care for the labor force scattered over California, Washington, and Oregon. At Richmond many workers remained only on regular workers' compensation because Permanente membership rolls were full. Garfield instituted two different health plans for workers at the Portland-Vancouver yards. One was Oregon Physicians' Service (OPS), formed by state medical society doctors in 1942 to meet the demands of war industry. The other was the Kaiser Permanente program. At the Oregon and Swan shipyards in Oregon, the Kaiser organization contracted with OPS in August 1942. Industrial care was compensated through the Oregon State Industrial Commission, and nonindustrial services were prepaid by employees for the sixty cents a week the company deducted from each worker's wages. That an estimated 65 percent of the eligible work force signed up for OPS at the two Oregon yards signified the critical need for medical care rather than enthusiasm for OPS.

Portland hospitals were overcrowded. The Kaiser company, with the USMC as prime contractor, finally built a 130-bed hospital at Vanport in the summer of 1943 staffed with two residents and one or two interns. It was open to all licensed physicians, but OPS controlled their access. Constructed as an infirmary, it was neither a financial nor medical success. Despite the shortage of beds in the area, and with over 37,000 residents in Vanport, the hospital stayed only about 60 percent full. It was not fully equipped; there was no prepayment plan for dependents, and even though there were many sick children in Vanport, the hospital was not able to care for them. In its first few months OPS suffered deficits up to $15,000 a month.

The health plan set up in Vancouver, Washington, was operated directly by the Northern Permanente Foundation and was based at the Northern Permanente Hospital designed by Garfield and financed by Kaiser and the USMC. The Permanente Foundation had a contract with the state of Washington, Department of Labor and Industries, to cover treatment and care of employees for industrial injuries.

Kaiser also had a family plan at Vancouver. For an additional sixty cents a week for the employee, thirty cents for a spouse, and fifteen cents per child, workers received comprehensive care for domestic illness and injury as well. Kaiser officials reported that the Vancouver plan was much more popular with labor than was the OPS plan in Oregon. Enrollment was much higher than it was for OPS, with 87 percent of the work force signed up by the end of 1943. One of Garfield's colleagues analyzed the reasons for the greater success at Vancouver. Though OPS paid physicians $500 a month (Kaiser paid $450 to $1,000 furnishing uniforms and all equipment.[33] The physicians and staff who worked directly for Garfield were younger and more dedicated to community welfare. The military depleted the supply of draft-age physicians, resulting in high demand for those who remained in private practice. By the end of 1943, the average age of the full-time OPS physicians had risen to sixty-five, while Kaiser's influence with national officials enabled him to gain deferments for essential young physicians.

Kaiser officials emphasized Garfield's ability to recruit a younger and more energetic medical staff. "Permanente men help in problems of employee and industry regardless of coverage," a supervising physician claimed, while OPS doctors refused to extend services or concern beyond a strict interpretation of the service contract. "Oregon Physicians' Service is not particularly concerned with the welfare of the people in the community," the report concluded.[34] The implication was that physician recruits were drawn to Permanente by an idealistic sense of community involvement that set them apart from their professional colleagues. They also were indirectly on the Kaiser payroll through their contracts with Garfield and Associates and did usually gain draft exempt status.

Despite a successful membership campaign, and the enormous growth of Kaiser Permanente, labor turnover and absenteeism remained at critical levels in all the West Coast shipyards. At first this was a result of lack of housing and poor living conditions. The company blamed later turnover on the military draft and poor health of those women, young people, older men, and military rejects left to work. The administrative difficulties of training half a million workers when only a fraction of them remained to work long-term were a tremendous burden on management.[35]

Turnover reached 15 percent monthly in Portland-Vancouver by mid-1943, and once shot as high as 150 percent. Observers blamed abominable living conditions. Franklin D. Roosevelt issued an executive order in early April 1943 to create a President's Committee for Congested Production Areas in an attempt to coordinate federal programs and ease housing, manpower, and goods and services shortages in those places hardest hit. These efforts helped to effect a decline in turnover, down to 7 percent the following year.[36] But workers suffered from poor living and sanitation facilities throughout the war.

In addition to the poor and often squalid living conditions, management at Richmond tied problems to the special character of the migrant workers brought by Kaiser, the majority from the South and Midwest. A hiring hall study revealed the negative conditions of travel and the chaotic circumstances upon arrival. The railroad companies failed to provide adequate food and accommodations in what the workers called "cattle cars" where they had to spend three or four days traveling. They arrived at Richmond in a "despondent mood," with nerves and bodies too weak to cope with the new difficulties they met on arrival. These "difficulties" were called the "run-around" by personnel officials, "magnified" by the lack of rest and nourishment. Standing in line at the information desk, the housing desk, the union, and the various departments proved overwhelming for new recruits, who also became discouraged by the damp climate and living conditions. Many sent home for money to return or "just drift on."[37]

Poor health was more characteristic of recruits from the South than from other groups. The hiring hall report speculated that this was caused by a deficiency of vitamin B_1, because heart conditions and similar ailments were common. Moreover, southerners suffered from syphilis at a rate 4 times the average in the North; blacks were infected 5.7 times more frequently than white workers.[38] The shipyard medical program did not treat ailments such as alcoholism, despondence, and other special problems of the recruits. Typical of insurance coverage of the era, Kaiser excluded insanity, alcoholism, drug addiction, venereal disease, attempts at suicide, "injuries resulting from professional boxing and wrestling," and any condition such as tuberculosis "that is active or manifestly existent" at the time the employee first signed up for coverage. Pregnancy "or conditions arising therefrom" was excluded in the same category as venereal disease and insanity.[39] These limits reflected the moralistic attitude toward public health carried over from the previous century and also preserved the financial health of the medical plan.

The Permanente Foundation and physicians were trailblazers, however, in the research and application of new antibiotics for treating diseases such as syphilis, gonorrhea, and pneumonia. Within months of the discovery of penicillin as a cure for syphilis and gonorrhea in early 1943 by Dr. John Mahoney of the U.S. Public Health Service, Permanente sent staff to Chicago for training to establish a syphilis clinic. Penicillin treatment for both venereal diseases replaced older fever therapy and was given to over 100 patients a month in early 1944. When women became a significant part of the work force, obstetrical care was offered, though later, during the postwar baby boom, for an extra charge of $25. Also the Permanente Foundation initiated special projects and treatment programs in pulmonary diseases. The treatment of tuberculosis in returning veterans was the major feature of the

Vancouver program. In northern California, Collen directed extensive statistical research. He combined sulfa and penicillin treatment for pneumonia in spite of objections by the conservative insurance companies and scarcity due to military demands.[40]

White southerners were a special problem for reasons other than their medical needs. They complained that "the shipyards employ, and they must mingle with, all races, creeds, and colors." Discrimination among workers and by the AFL locals was a persistent problem for Kaiser, both at the Portland-Vancouver yards and in the Bay Area. The first great migration of black workers to the West during the early 1940s thrust racial issues into prominence in labor-management relations.[41]

Because federal contracts were the foundation of the Kaiser industrial empire, the corporation closely adhered to federal employment regulations. The industrialist's son and top manager, Edgar Kaiser, prided himself on social liberalism, but his early closed-shop master's agreement with the discriminatory metal trades unions greatly tarnished his image among black activists and the Fair Employment Practices Commission (FEPC) established by presidential order. In 1942 Kaiser recruiters in the East avoided hiring black workers, allowing the AFL New York Building Trades Council to place their order for 20,000 shipyard workers with the U.S. Employment Service. The council acted as a "clearing house to sort out black recruits," according to one historian. Edgar Kaiser admitted that black workers were a problem for the company because of the lack of housing for them in the larger community. The company constructed thousands of dormitory units specifically for these residents unwanted in white working-class society. That their stay in the region was considered temporary might explain why they made up a disproportionate 20 percent of Vanport residents when they were only 7.2 percent of the Kaiser work force of more than 84,000 in 1944.[42]

Local housing authority studies indicated a more deliberate move toward racially segregated housing in Richmond and Oakland that laid the groundwork for the postwar patchwork pattern of segregated housing that became permanent. Richmond and the harbor front areas in Oakland became "overnight migrant ghettos." The Oakland Housing Authority segregated blacks in the Harbor Homes project in Oakland near the Moore shipyards. In Richmond, housing officials placed blacks near the shipyards and railroads in shoreline areas. The outlying residential tiers were all white, acting as a buffer for established residents. An informal quota system used by the Federal Public Housing Authority (FPHA) during the war was applied in Richmond at a ratio of four to one in 1943. With only 20 percent of residential units allotted to blacks, families had to move in together, creating overcrowded housing and a network of illegal sublets. A January 1945 survey found that 80 out of 360 black families but only 16 of 3,500 white families were in illegal housing arrangements. After the war segregated housing spread from the war projects along the waterfront on the southern and eastern edges to create an all-black settlement pattern on the southside by the 1960s. The same process happened at Hunters Point, Marin City, Vallejo, and other war boom towns in the San Francisco Bay Area.[43]

Thus, Kaiser war industries permanently altered the urban landscape of the region, as well as its social welfare institutions. Kaiser Permanente was the core of the Bay Area health system and a symbol of the new community order. Kaiser industries and the health plan counteracted the negative attitudes toward rapid population changes expressed by local government. The Welfare Council of Richmond charged in a highly prejudicial postwar report that war housing residents had "no feeling of participation in the life of the city, no sense of responsibility as citizens . . . for the welfare and future of the city as a whole."[44] They were treated as temporary residents.

Black residents were actively discriminated against. During public hearings in 1943, complainants reported that the Kaiser Corporation discharged 300 black workers from the Portland yard in the last two weeks of July, and 165 skilled black workers from the San Francisco Bay Area yards. Edgar Kaiser was frustrated. He was caught between federal labor regulations to honor the AFL closed-shop agreement, and union demands that the company fire blacks for not paying dues to the union auxiliaries they were forced to join as second-class members. Soon the unions turned on Kaiser, accusing the company of "foot-dragging" on demands to fire blacks for not paying dues.[45]

While Kaiser was criticized for not confronting AFL racism, there is no evidence that blacks were discriminated against in Kaiser medical facilities. Black workers eventually represented 14.5 percent of the work force at Richmond, and almost 20 percent in Vancouver, and no overt instances of discrimination were reported. Nor is there a record of subtle racism occurring among individual patients and staff. A Kaiser official recalled that the shipyard medical facilities and health plan were fully integrated, and hence that Permanente hospitals did not suffer the protests made against other California health care institutions after the war by civil rights activists. In 1945, when the health plan opened to public enrollment, the left-wing CIO ILWU hailed Permanente as "open to all groups with no segregation of patients because of creed or color."[46]

Against the obstructions of labor shortages, turnover, absenteeism, and internecine labor disputes, Kaiser triumphed. Efficient recruitment and use of manpower cut production time to forty-six days per ship by mid-1942, beating the USMC deadline by ninety-four days and making Kaiser a national war hero. Furthermore, the overall safety record of the Richmond yards was impressive. In 1942 the USMC cited Kaiser as having the lowest loss ratio of injuries, sickness, and time loss to productive man hours of any war industry in California.[47]

Kaiser health planners supported concepts of holistic preventive care. They wanted subscribers to have the feeling "that this plan is their own and that the entire staff are working towards providing them with the best medical attention possible." They emphasized nutrition. The staff surveyed the San Francisco Bay Area workers and found that at least 60 percent did not have "adequate breakfasts" and often were unable to get adequate lunches at the job site. A memo widely distributed in April 1943 to key doctors and managers also noted a newly emergent problem—the changing profile of Kaiser workers. By 1944 female workers were 25 percent of the Kaiser labor force; 30 percent more were men over the draft age. Still other men were younger, but with physical disabilities. With so many female, elderly, and disabled workers, the memo recommended that "extra consideration should be given for handling the cases of the undernourished as well as ladies and elderly men." The suggestion was made to develop a hot lunch plan and dispense vitamins at the workers' expense, so that "more value would be placed upon their use." Management hoped to "bring about greater vitality, greater psychological effect and consequently increased productivity."[48]

Generally, however, government agencies addressed community and family needs, leaving occupational care to Kaiser. Accustomed to speaking of "working men," Kaiser failed to emphasize in his comments on the health plan and other aspects of his operations the growing dependence on women workers. The Richmond shipyard weekly magazine, *Fore 'N' Aft*, announced the hiring of the first ten women welders in the July 1942 issue. Two years later women were 27.5 percent of all Richmond shipyard employees. At the peak of female employment, there were 24,500 women on the Richmond payroll. Workers and Kaiser officials recognized that the pressures of household and childrearing responsibilities greatly increased anxiety and physical hardship for women and were the reason for their higher absentee and turnover rate. Absenteeism at Portland-Vancouver fluctuated from 11 to over 13 percent for women, while for men it was between 7 and 9 percent. Though living conditions generally were better than at Richmond, and absenteeism lower, women there also suffered from inadequate provisions for child care and other necessities connected with family life. One cartoon in the shipyard's newspaper depicted a distraught and angry woman with a burning pot in the background, holding a pan to heat a baby bottle in one hand while thrusting the telephone receiver at her screaming children with the other. The caption read: "Here [to her infant], you talk to the foreman. Explain why I didn't show up for work today."[49]

Though one author emphasizes that a "sexual division of labor" persisted, with women remaining in the "helper" and unskilled categories, women did receive equal wages for doing the same work as men. Domestic amenities such as child care centers at the workplace were extolled by Eleanor Roosevelt, and precooked meals that could be taken home also facilitated employment. Using USMC funds Kaiser corporation created two large "child service centers" in Portland that cost parents $5.00 a week for one child and $3.75 for the second child, ages eighteen months to six years.[50] The centers reached their highest enrollment figures in the summer of 1944, with 444 children at Swan Island and 390 at Oregon Shipbuilding. Even though women workers had to pay weekly fees to use the centers, they were enormously popular.[51]

Kaiser's child care program at Portland-Vancouver was nationally acclaimed, but like the medical program it had strong critics alienated by Kaiser's usurpation of traditional spheres of authority in U.S. culture. The War Manpower Commission held the position that "the first responsibility of women with young children in war as in peace is to give suitable care to their children." Community committees organized to address the growing problem of women with young children on the production lines. The Portland *Oregonian* warned of the increase in juvenile delinquency and quoted a city health officer as saying that "many mothers apparently prefer $60 a week now to good health and behavior for their children later."[52]

City agencies sought to prevent employment of women with children under age fourteen. But the community could not handle the production emergency and fast-escalating entry of women into the work force. By March 1943 830 mothers of preschool children already worked for Kaiser. In May the industrialist announced plans for three nurseries, one at each shipyard, each for 450 children. They were funded by the USMC rather than with the Lanham Act funds that would require local day-care committee approval, which Kaiser did not have. Multnomah County, Vancouver, and the state of Oregon opposed them, as did the U.S. Office of Education, the U.S. Children's Bureau, the women advisors of the USMC, and the Oregon State Medical Society. These groups

organized opposition to Kaiser child care because it encouraged the mothers of young children to work outside of home.[53]

Social welfare leaders objected to the employer's involvement in child care with the same rationale that the AMA used
to voice objection to contract practice and company involvement in the intimate recesses of family medical life. Industry's
concern was production, not the welfare of children, opponents argued. Kaiser bucked tradition on the question of
working mothers just as he did on other community health
and welfare issues. He said in a *New York Times* interview in
October 1943 that "factories should be equipped with child-
care centers, health clinics, shopping centers, food dispensers,
banking facilities, dry cleaning shops, recreation centers, com-
fortable lockers and rest rooms" in what he called "the factory
of the future."[54]

Kaiser built two child care centers in Portland without local
approval, but bowed to local authorities at Vancouver, where
Lanham funds were used by the Clark County Child Care
Committee. Edgar Kaiser regained the trust of the social welfare network by turning to the best experts in the country to
staff and direct the centers. Moreover, Eleanor Roosevelt was
an outspoken champion of the effort. Urging Admiral Emory
Land, chair of the USMC, to give the Kaisers permission to
build the centers, she expressed support for working women
well ahead of traditional mores. "I have long known that the
only way we could possibly get the women that we need to take
jobs was to provide them with community services," she wrote.
"If the shipbuilding companies will recognize this fact, that it
is a part of being able to do their jobs to render these services,
it may spread to other industries and will help enormously in
war production."[55]

But the Kaiser organization did not seek long-term solutions to the problems of working mothers. New York reformer and philanthropist Albert D. Lasker congratulated
Henry Kaiser for approving the distribution of birth control
information in the Permanente clinics; at the same time, child-
birth was not covered in the Permanente Health Plan when it
first was established. Benefits for "female employees who enter the hospital for maternity nine months or more after their

insurance becomes effective, and within nine months after termination of insurance" were not advertised until mid-1944. Women were considered only a temporary part of the work force, in accordance with conventional mores. Kaiser publicists emphasized women's domestic role. To "put aside the welder's torch" and return to the kitchen was the working woman's goal.[56] Nevertheless, the company gradually relaxed the moral and sexist restrictions of its health plan. It needed to attract married women workers whose husbands were off to war. Kaiser assured them that maternity benefits would be a benefit of employment that they could cash in at war's end when they left work to raise families.

A vital legacy of the shipyard experience for Kaiser was that the large number of women workers showed him that corporations would in the future need to take responsibility for worker family care. Local doctors at Richmond trying to function with a doctor-patient ratio of 1 to 7,000 were unable to give adequate care to family members. Often no hospital beds were available, and physicians were forced to open wards in dark and ill-equipped hospital basements. Family care in the midst of the population explosion became as much a headache for Kaiser planners as for the local medical establishment. Kaiser and Garfield said in Senate committee testimony at the end of 1942 that they were unable to provide family care because of threats to draft Kaiser doctors by the AMA-controlled Procurement and Assignment Service. But Henry Kaiser also admitted that Kaiser Permanente did not have the capability to provide care for families in 1942 and 1943, beyond the limited hospital plans at Vancouver and for about 3,500 workers at Fontana. Like Richmond, the Fontana plan was often closed to new members. Kaiser called the medical society restriction of further expansion to families "satisfactory."[57]

The U.S. Public Health Service fulfilled a traditional role in the shipyard communities, policing sanitation problems and unhealthy behavior. The problems of the overcrowded and unsanitary material environment were exacerbated by habits such as improper garbage disposal and sexual promiscuity.

The *Fortune* magazine feature of the Richmond yards appearing in early 1945 displayed typical moral biases of the era in its sympathetic portrayal of the public spiritedness of Kaiser, city government, and federal agencies in caring for the uneducated and indigent migrant working class. The reporter wrote that despite the small PHS staff of three Red Cross nurses, eleven public health nurses, three clinic doctors, and five sanitary inspectors, and despite poor conditions in the yard, the "closest thing to an epidemic" were fifty cases of poliomyelitis in 1943. There was also a "high rate" of venereal disease and tuberculosis in men and women "doing unusually hard work." The state and PHS ran clinics for those afflicted with these ailments, traditionally not covered by any type of private insurance or industrial health plan. The service also claimed to take on care of dependents for the 87 percent of the work force who joined the Kaiser Health Plan. It provided immunization, as well as care for "crippled children" and "well babies." It recorded 1,800 births in 1944, but *Fortune*'s moralizing echoed that of the Richmond Welfare Committee: "At least three out of four of these babies were born into temporary, precarious surroundings, to parents with no ties to the land, no roots in the community."[58]

Kaiser's decision in 1944 to continue the medical program after the war, and to offer it to the general public, necessitated a full-fledged commitment to family health to attract members outside the Kaiser shipyards. Garfield experimented with a health plan for civilian employees at the Harbor Gate federal housing project in the East Bay against county medical society opposition. Kaiser planners did considerable juggling of cost per family and benefits to assure economic viability. The FHA imposed difficult demands. There was a moralistic tinge to agency charges of "ambiguous wording" in Kaiser's member agreement and of an attempt to "draw a line through a homogeneous family group" by excluding from the family rate children over eighteen living at home and those under eighteen who were employed. Federal officials wanted the monthly subscription rate for family coverage dropped from the $7.50 originally proposed by Garfield to $5.00. They compromised on $1.60 a week, or $6.40 a month for a family of four, considerably more than the $4.80 a Kaiser worker paid at the Vancouver shipyards for family membership, reflecting corporate trepidation at unknown variables when the health plan was extended outside corporate territory.[59]

Yet the plan still was a tremendous bargain for working-class families. A 1944 survey by the United Steelworkers found that their members spent an average of $10.82 a month or $129.84 a year per family for medical care that was neither preventive nor comprehensive. This represented about 5 percent of an average annual income of $2,584.[60] At $76.80 a year, families at Harbor Gate with the same income were spending about 3 percent for comprehensive health care.

Kaiser's intention to extend the prepaid group plan to families in the larger community after the war was evident in a number of early public pronouncements by the industrialist. In 1942, at hospital dedication ceremonies at Oakland, Kaiser expressed a vision for the future. Announcing the creation of the Permanente Foundation, Kaiser stated its threefold purpose: to "provide funds for research in industrial medicine"; "set up fellowships for the training of physicians and nurses in specialties"; and build modern facilities to induce young doctors coming out of the military to go into group practice, serving those heretofore deprived of adequate medical care. Kaiser's vision echoed CCMC proposals for large-scale regional group practice and regional planning. He thus aped the elite intellectual blueprint for a national health system, and the traditions of the Rockefeller and Carnegie foundations for research and education.[61]

Material expansion demonstrated Kaiser's success. The Permanente Foundation financed four hospitals for shipyard and Fontana steel plant workers during the war. They included the Vancouver Northern Permanente Foundation Hospital with 339 beds and thirty doctors' offices, and the renovated Oakland Permanente Foundation Hospital with 300 beds and fifty doctors' offices. The 100-bed Richmond Field Hospital remained, along with the 50-bed Fontana hospital with five offices. After the war the foundation bought out the government's share of facilities, undertaking an expansion program in the next decade that reached $12 million.[62]

By the end of July 1945 about 50,000 workers had left the Kaiser yards in northern California. Health plan membership dwindled to about 7,500 in the San Francisco Bay Area, and in all regions combined it was only 17,000. Garfield and Associates aggressively sought outside client groups. These included the residents of Harbor Gate where the family plan was first offered, and civilian employees of the Naval Air Station at Alameda. Permanente started small clinics in Vallejo and Napa for federal civil service maritime workers. Cutting took over an Industrial Indemnity insurance clinic in San Francisco where the Kaiser plan already had a substantial wartime membership. Within six months after the plan was offered to the public in July 1945, membership was 26,000. Within a decade it grew twentyfold to well over half a million members. The majority were employee and union groups, which propelled rapid expansion of the medical program outward from the three wartime Kaiser production sites at Portland-Vancouver, Richmond, and Fontana.[63] The most dramatic expansion occurred in southern California, centered in the Los Angeles metropolitan area.

Kaiser's health plan in northern California was a matrix of the new regional culture, the receptacle of an abstract definition of a community of shared experiences and values attained during the war. It sustained a voluntary communitarian bond, manifest internally as an insular medical practice culture shared by Permanente physicians. The holistic social values of this culture were disseminated in the physicians' interactions with members and patients in the larger regional community, as former shipyard workers dispersed along the urban coast.

Garfield later said that he "didn't see the unions coming into our operations, but it couldn't be avoided." Also, he "didn't like the idea that the people themselves weren't paying for the health plan" because they would be lax about their own health.[64] His remarks reflected a power shift in labor-capital relations first set in motion by New Deal welfare legislation and the formation of the CIO in 1935. The most permanent gain of the labor movement in the 1930s and 1940s was what John R. Commons first labeled a system of "private social security" through collective bargaining. Its keystone was health and retirement benefits encouraged by government programs and legislation. In 1942 the War Labor Board ruled that such benefits up to 5 percent of wages were not inflationary and were tax deductible. Employers increased them to aid in recruitment and to solidify employee loyalty during the wartime labor shortage. Employer tax incentives were continued by the Revenue Act of 1945.

Union leaders seized the advantage in the mixed public and private welfare state that emerged. Their authority in collective bargaining for welfare benefits increased the loyalty of the rank and file to the unions. At the same time it diminished the loyalty companies had formerly garnered through welfare capitalism.[65] Yet Henry Kaiser retained the esteem of U.S. workers that fellow industrial capitalists lost to militant labor leaders, retaining paternalistic authority in the working-class community through his health plan.

By the end of the first year of public operation, only 15 percent of Permanente Health Plan members in northern California were Kaiser employees. The California CIO and AFL Alameda County Central Labor Council both recommended the Kaiser plan to members, who joined at the rate of 2,000 a month. The *East Bay Labor Journal* extolled the principle of preventive medicine practiced by Permanente. The first AFL affiliates included Bay Area locals of the Milk Wagon Drivers, Oakland Typographical Union, Office Employees' International, Building Service Employees, and Cleaning and Dye House Workers unions.[66]

The Bay Area was an AFL stronghold, but leftist CIO locals also joined Permanente, including the ILWU, United Electrical Workers (UE) Local 1412, and the Federation of Architects, Engineers, Chemists and Technicians, Chapter 25. In July 1945, it was the only health plan the state CIO council endorsed.

The ILWU press recommended the Kaiser plan in June 1945 as part of all future negotiations for benefits with employers in the San Francisco Bay Area. Local 6 vice-president Paul Heide told members that Kaiser had "unusual medical facilities, not ordinarily available to individual practicing physicians" for the cost of sixty cents a week for men and seventy-five cents for women. If state insurance went into effect, as union officials desired, the Permanente Hospital "would be blanketed under the act and no money would be lost by members who join it now." The principle of preventive medicine made Permanente superior, union spokespersons said, to the California Physician's Service plan. By mid-October Longshoremen's Local 10 members were enrolling through a payroll deduction of $2.60 a month, with dependents eligible at reduced rates.[67]

The ILWU epitomized the regional changes in ethnic demography embodied by Kaiser membership. Black longshoremen from the Gulf coast migrated west during World War II as German submarines curtailed eastern shipping. As the shipyards laid off tens of thousands of workers in 1944 and 1945, men of every race came to the docks for employment. One-fifth of the 2,600 San Pedro recruits between July 1944 and July 1945 were black, even though a few white members earlier sought to keep them out. The 3,100 new workers in Seattle included a small proportion of blacks, though the Portland local maintained its traditional white profile. In Portland black workers suffered the same prejudices they had faced from the Boilermakers' union in the Kaiser shipyards.

There was a profound racial transformation of Bay Area ILWU Local 10. Of 6,600 new members in the last year of the war, nearly half were former black shipyard workers. At the end of 1945 the local was nearly one-third black. Moreover, the union was far to the left on the national political spectrum, its white and black members discriminated against equally in the anti-Communist reactionism that erupted on the waterfront in May 1950. The Coast Guard denied work passes for military docks to 243 longshoremen in San Francisco. Two-thirds of them were black, according to a union survey. A few weeks later the CIO expelled the union from its ranks, along with ten other unions, for suspected Communist influence. In 1939, the U.S. government had begun a series of efforts to deport longshoremen organizer Harry Bridges to his native Australia.[68]

Of the thirty-five CIO unions nationwide in 1946, historians estimate that twelve had Communist-inspired leadership. Another twelve had alleged Communists in leadership positions, including the ILWU and UE. With half a million members, the UE was the largest of the suspect unions.

Although they had far fewer numbers, the Mine, Mill and Smelter Workers (later the United Steelworkers) at the western reclamation projects in the 1930s, and the ILWU in the late 1940s and early 1950s, were aggressive unions that influenced Kaiser Permanente program development. Both were leftist unions in vital industries. The Steelworkers' locals in California were a natural Kaiser plan constituency. The 3,000 workers at Fontana who already had the benefit of a comprehensive medical program with Kaiser that included families remained members after the war. In northern California the Bethlehem Pacific Coast Steel Company local in South San Francisco selected the Kaiser plan, and Local 1440 at the U.S. Steel Corporation's Columbia Geneva plant in Pittsburg, California, expressed interest in Kaiser. During massive strikes in 1946 and 1947 in the steel, mine, and railroad industries, the San Francisco local entered arbitration with the steel company to decide whether labor or management would select health coverage. The union won the dispute.[69]

The Kaiser plan expanded from the three wartime production sites at a highly uneven rate. Membership in northern California grew at a fast and steady pace from the shipyard labor base and stayed under the immediate purview of corporate headquarters in Oakland. The Northwest program at Portland and Vancouver got off to a slow and shaky start. Dr. Ernest W. Saward joined the program in June 1945 as assistant to Grand Coulee veteran Wallace Neighbor and soon replaced Neighbor as Northern Permanente medical director. Saward had been medical director at the government-owned uranium and plutonium facility at Hanford, Washington. Ordway perhaps discovered him, as he had Garfield on the southern California desert, when he was in Hanford to oversee Kaiser engineering contracts.

The Northwest program was financially insolvent in the early years, and independent patient fees, along with a contract with the Veterans Administration (VA) to care for tuberculosis patients, were all that kept it afloat. It remained the slowest growing region, and Saward complained of the paucity of material allocations and lack of interest by the Kaiser trustees, with the exception of Edgar Kaiser who raised his family in the area. In 1946 Edgar left to oversee the Kaiser-Frazer automobile plant in Michigan.

After the war Northern Permanente retained only the Vancouver Hospital. In 1948 the formerly bustling company town of Vanport was washed away by a flood. The location and physical condition of the hospital discouraged membership growth. Most shipyard workers who remained to find new employment after the war moved to the Portland side of the river to work for other employers. Regional membership dwindled to 3,000, less than the tiny Fontana.

Saward sought the veteran's contract for men chronically ill with tuberculosis as a solution to the financial crisis at the 300-bed, largely empty hospital. Streptomycin was the first effective antibiotic against the disease, available by 1947, and Saward claimed his hospital was one of the first to use it widely. The patients had psychological problems as well. Many were prisoners of war held by the Japanese for four years. Relieved of strict military confinement for the first time, they literally ran wild. Saward observed that "they did any damn thing they wanted." He constantly had to bail them out of jail, a fairly easy matter since local jailers did not want responsibility. "They would disappear," he said. "We would try and find them. Some of them were murdered. They'd get in the damnedest scrapes." Saward was a social medicine and public health ideologue who exemplified the early leadership in Permanente's unorthodox medical culture. The American Hospital Association reported that few hospitals were willing to participate in the VA program of arranging care for service-disabled veterans in their home communities. They had to be sent to remote facilities.[70] Their reputation and neglect echoed that of the turbulent and rootless seamen of the previous century. Saward scrambled for the government contract to care for this neglected patient population, and the Portland-Vancouver program survived because it provided care for a group at the bottom of the socioeconomic scale under government sponsorship.

The Northwest's Northern Permanente plan also had support from local colleges and public press, typically liberal institutions. In 1945 the Reed College faculty was one of the first new member groups, as were the new Vanport College (now Portland State College) faculty and the *Oregonian* newspaper staff. Health plan representative Avram Yedidia emphasized the support of academic institutions in northern California as well, including the University of California, Mills College, and San Francisco State University. Their liberal influence complemented that of the ILWU and other left-wing unions. Combined with the increasing numbers of state and federal employee groups, the large liberal constituency added cohesion to a progressive integration policy at Permanente facilities.[71] The Portland-Vancouver region continued to develop at a much less dramatic pace than the California regions. The problem of location persisted until the Bess Kaiser Hospital was built in Portland in 1959, honoring Henry Kaiser's first wife.

Southern California expansion from the tiny Fontana embryo was the most dramatic example of union-prompted growth in the postwar decade. Although it did not take off until 1950, it then grew 193 percent within five years. By 1955, health plan membership was 301,671 in northern California, 199,043 in southern California, and only 22,796 in the Northwest.[72]

Harry Bridges and Joe DeSilva, president of the AFL Retail Clerks' Union Local 70, first urged Kaiser to move the medical program outside the plant gates at Fontana. Kaiser and his top adviser, Eugene (Gene) Trefethen, resisted. "The people up here [in the Bay Area] just did not like southern California," Garfield explained. Nevertheless, in 1949 Garfield made Raymond Kay medical director at Fontana under a separate plan he called the Sidney R. Garfield and Associates Health Plan, opened to the public. Until then Kay supplemented his income by teaching for three years after the war at the Los Angeles County Hospital and the University of Southern California, as Garfield had before him.[73]

In early 1950 the ILWU officially asked Garfield to take on all its unionized ports, 22,510 members. The largest group was in the San Francisco Bay Area ports, with about 6,300 families with an average of 2.5 dependents. The following year DeSilva asked the Kaiser trustees to develop a family medical program for about 26,500 retail clerks (Local 770) in greater Los Angeles; 85.5 percent chose to join Kaiser. About 22,000 culinary workers also joined in southern California. The union enrollment included families averaging 2.5 dependents. Garfield in a 1984 interview did not express an opinion about Bridges but said he got along easily with De-Silva, calling him "Mr. Kaiser on a smaller scale." "He really liked us," Garfield recalled.[74]

The full health plan went into effect for union members in San Francisco, Los Angeles, and Portland-Vancouver on 1 February 1950, under the coastwide welfare plan signed by the union with Pacific Maritime Associates (PMA) as a supplement to the Pacific Coast Longshore Agreement. Comprehensive prepaid group service plans soon covered 80 percent of members.

Garfield went to great lengths to satisfy the ILWU. Union membership in the Kaiser Health Plan was the basis for regional expansion outside the San Francisco Bay Area. Since Permanente was not available at all ports, Garfield helped the union set up contracts with three smaller prepaid group plans. The largest was the Group Health Cooperative of Puget Sound, based in Seattle. By 1953 Group Health covered about 2,000 workers at $10 a month, including families. The other two plans, at $8 a month, were the Coos Bay Hospital Association, serving about 1,300 people in three Oregon ports, and Grays Harbor Community Hospital for 360 members and dependents at the port ILWU local at Aberdeen, Washington. The fourth option was for indemnity coverage with New York Life Insurance for about 10,000 persons scattered the length of the coast with carefully itemized coverage at $11.55 a month. Garfield thus organized medical care for a total of 35,605 members under the ILWU-PMA benefit program

TABLE 2.1. Health Plan Membership for Selected Dates,
1945–1958

Date	Northern Calif.	Southern Calif.	Portland/ Vancouver	Total
1945	11,500	—	15,000	26,500
1950	120,000	20,000	14,000	154,000
1951	160,000	67,000	17,000	244,000
1952	188,000	76,000	19,000	283,000
Jan. 1953	191,000	54,000/[a] 23,000	20,000	288,000
July 1953	213,000	105,000/ 22,000	21,000	361,000
Dec. 1953	240,000	115,000/ 25,000	22,000	402,000
Jan. 1954	241,000	126,000/ 24,000	22,000	413,000
July 1954	266,000	140,000/ 25,000	22,000	453,000
Dec. 1954	278,000	149,000 28,000	22,000	477,000
Jan. 1955	282,000	150,000/ 29,000	22,000	483,000
June 1955	291,000	158,000/ 30,000	22,000	501,000
Dec. 1955	302,000	199,000	23,000	524,000
1956	315,000	218,000	23,000	556,000

TABLE 2.1. (Continued)

Date	Northern Calif.	Southern Calif.	Portland/ Vancouver	Total
1957	317,000	234,000	24,000	575,000
1958	337,000	245,000	30,000	618,000

SOURCE: "Table, Health Plan Membership for Selected Years," carton 339; "Kaiser Foundation Health Plan Membership as at December 31st for the Years 1950 to 1963," carton 247; "Total Health Plan Membership, January 1953–June 1955 [with percentages]," carton 117, HJK Papers.
NOTE: The Hawaii Region opened on 15 November 1958 with 6,000 members. By 1960 it had 38,616 members.
^{a}First figure is for Los Angeles, second for Fontana.

jointly with the employers' association. The ILWU contract ignited Kaiser's membership explosion from about 8,500 to 20,000 in a single year in southern California. Within a year of gaining their own welfare package in 1953, about 4,000 members joined Kaiser from the warehouse locals.[75]

At Portland-Vancouver the ILWU boosted the Northwest program just as the veterans' contract terminated. Longshoremen of Portland Port Local 8 and their dependents joined in early 1950. The 4,710 ILWU members, with an average of four family members, according to Saward, raised group enrollment by 21 percent in the first two years. By 1954, the ILWU represented almost one-fourth of total Kaiser membership in the region.[76] At the end of 1954 the northern California health plan had over 14,000 ILWU members and 30,000 Culinary Workers, including their dependents. These two unions alone made up 16 percent of Kaiser membership in the region. In southern California the ILWU and the Retail Clerks and Culinary Workers unions, with their families, represented one-third of regional membership.[77]

Until contracts were signed with the dominant union groups after 1950, in the first two years of public operation most Permanente enrollment was on an individual, self-pay basis. Public employees at the municipal, state, and federal levels were a large membership contingent in northern California. An enterprising administrator, Al Brodie, instituted a federal collectors' program. Representatives from small enclaves of federal workers volunteered to collect dues and administer health plan membership. Brodie received about a nickel a month per subscriber for his efforts, and the individual collector also took a small percentage, in addition to pro bono health plan coverage. In this way, thousands joined, including about a thousand families of San Francisco municipal employees in 1948 when local doctors withdrew from the Health Service System. Kaiser membership henceforth increased steadily among city workers. Thousands in United Auto Workers (UAW) and Steelworkers' locals also began self-administered plans with Kaiser. By 1951 in northern California 900 union and employee groups provided the bulk of membership (see tables 2.1 and 2.2).[78]

TABLE 2.2. Representative Health Plan Groups, March 1951
San Francisco Bay Area

Group[a]	Number of Family Units[b]
ILWU-PMA Welfare Fund	6,300
Mare Island Naval Shipyard	3,256
Naval Air Station, Alameda	1,485
University of California	1,334
San Francisco Naval Shipyard, Hunter's Point	1,319
Kaiser Employees	864
Carpenters Union Locals 1158, 1149, 642, 36, and 1622	826
Bethlehem Steel Co., S. San Francisco	640
United Office and Professional Workers of America	565
East Bay Cooperative Medical Group	493
Moore Dry Dock Co.	365
California Cotton Mills	336
U.S. Postal Employees, Oakland	300
H. C. Capwell Co.	270
Automotive Mechanics Union	248
Richmond School Dept.	248

TABLE 2.2. (Continued)

Group[a]	Number of Family Units[b]
Emporium, San Francisco	243
Colgate-Palmolive-Peet Co.	233
International Harvester Co.	213
National Automotive Fibres, Inc.	203
Typographical Union	202
Milk Wagon Drivers Union	197
Durkee's Famous Foods	164
W. P. Fuller Co., S. San Francisco	160
Golden State Milk Co., Oakland	141
East Bay Municipal Utility District	137
Berkeley Schools	122
San Francisco State College	118
Rheem Manufacturing Co., Richmond	91
Hercules Powder Co., Pinole	88
Sherman Clay and Co., San Francisco and Oakland	84
El Dorado Oil Works	80
Office Employees International Union	67
Mills College	58
Church Divinity School of the Pacific	57
Borden's Dairy Delivery, Oakland	56

SOURCE: Booklet, *The Inside Story—The Permanente Health Plan and a Proposal for Los Angeles and San Francisco* (N.d., n.p., but probably ca. 1951, Oakland), carton 87:18, EFK Papers.
[a]These groups represent more than 900 employee groups, with approximately 75,474 members, or 62% of the northern California membership.
[b]Family units average 2.5 members.

Strong labor support of Kaiser Permanente on the West Coast fulfilled the prediction of Kaiser's growing national influence in health care in the magazines of publisher Henry Luce. A 1944 article in *Fortune* magazine entitled "U.S. Medicine in Transition" surmised that national health reform was inevitable because 90 percent of Americans could not afford care under the solo practice fee-for-service system. The choice before the public was compulsory federal indemnity insurance through legislation then before Congress, or a voluntary system that added group practice to the prepaid cooperative group plans then in existence. The author highlighted only three prepaid group practice plans: Ross-Loos, GHA, and Kaiser. In 1943 prepaid group plans still enrolled only 7.7 percent of all union members and less than 1.5 percent of the total population. The Kaiser shipyard plan was the largest. Nevertheless, the author concluded that the prepaid group practice cut down medical service costs by 30 percent and represented the onset of a structural "transition" in U.S. medicine. He urged doctors to support the new form of practice; otherwise they would trail in the wake of initiatives by consumer cooperatives, labor, and industry. In a subsequent *Fortune* article, Garfield pointed to preventive "maintenance of health" as the primary operating principle of the Kaiser plan.[79] As had public health ideologues at least two decades earlier, Garfield and Kaiser merged industrial medicine, public health, and free enterprise to create a model for national health maintenance.

Henry Kaiser began to emphasize the expansive quality of his medical program in 1942 Senate testimony and in correspondence with public officials. In a battle with the Alameda County Medical Association over facilities expansion in 1943, Kaiser wrote to Charles E. Wilson, vice-president of the War Production Board and future chair of General Motors: "I sincerely believe that someday you will be grateful for having had the opportunity to support this type of institution. I am sorry that your [local Urgency] committee complains of pressure from Washington, without recognizing that the greatest amount of destructive and not reliable pressure has come from physicians and hospitals who fail to visualize a new world, more filled with productive employment, and more and better medical care."[80]

3   The Politics
of National Health

Each enthusiastic, interested pioneer of such schemes [industrial health] dreams of seeing his plan grow until it supplies service to the whole community. They picture industrial medical service expanding until it includes all employees and their dependents. . . . They would have lodges or unions include the entire population.

—*AMA report*, Organized Payments of Medical Services

SIDNEY GARFIELD DEVELOPED THE MEDICAL PROGRAM in the Kaiser shipyards against a backdrop of political acrimony in the health care field. The traditional world of solo fee-for-service doctors was shaken in the early 1940s by a number of events, not the least of which was Kaiser's "new world" venture in health care for the U.S. worker. Social unrest, the stress of war, the roller-coaster economy, labor militancy, and the efforts of the Truman administration to extend the Democratic welfare state after Roosevelt's death set conservatives on the warpath against New Deal liberalism through the 1940s. The politics of national health became a battleground on which industrial capitalists, labor, the U.S. defense establishment, and liberal politicians allied against the AMA, representing the large majority of the country's physicians.

A statement by Garfield before the AMA's annual conference

in June 1944, a year before the Kaiser plan was offered to the public, suggests why Kaiser would become an AMA target. "We have a fundamental concept," he said. Occupational health and safety problems "are rapidly being eliminated and are actually minor problems superimposed on the general health problem of the worker and his family." The bounds of the corporate industrial health plan were limitless. "Industrial health actually resolves itself to be not an entity but the basic health of the American people."[1]

Threatened by loss of income and community status, doctors in the AMA affiliates in northern California tried to stop Kaiser physician draft deferment and facilities expansion. In October 1942 Dr. Cecil Cutting had an unpleasant conference with Dr. Harold Fletcher, chair of the U.S. Procurement and Assignment Service for the region, and a leader in the Alameda County Medical Association (ACMA). Fletcher told Cutting that he opposed the extension of prepaid group medical care into the housing projects then under discussion by Kaiser and the Federal Housing Authority, for civilian employees of the U.S. Navy. Kaiser family care was particularly onerous to local physicians because it invaded the domain of private practice.

Fletcher called Garfield's medical service "a concession of the Kaiser organization as a peanut stand." Though he knew it had the backing of the USMC as well as of Henry Kaiser, he charged that it was "like Mr. Kaiser, who has been ruthless in getting steel, going ahead single-handed and without giving a thought or consideration of the Procurement Board or the medical profession on the outside, and their ability to take care of the workmen." He thought that Garfield "went ahead and enticed other [medical] men to come in with the assurance of being deferred from the Army." Fletcher warned that "it would be unwise if Mr. Kaiser backed Dr. Garfield further than he already had." He also stated that Permanente doctors would not be admitted to the county medical societies. Fletcher concluded the meeting by declaring his antagonism against "corporation medicine of which this [Kaiser Permanente] is a type." He "thought the California Physicians' Service [CPS] and medical profession themselves should take care of the health of the workers."[2]

The West Coast county medical societies were among the first in the nation to create their own prepayment plans as a defense against the spread of contract practice and corporate medicine. These combined to comprise the state plans. CPS formed in 1939, attracting 5,000 of the 7,000 California physicians. It was the first statewide medical society–sponsored service plan, soon followed by the Michigan Medical Service and the Western New York Medical Plan. The Multnomah County Medical Society created the Oregon Physicians' Service in 1942, which contracted for care of Kaiser shipyard workers in Portland.

According to the AMA its county society affiliates were the cornerstone of professional organization and its first line of defense against outside competition. "The county medical society," the AMA asserted in 1939, "is the only organization occupying the national geographic unit and possessed of the necessary professional knowledge and the power to maintain the Principles of Medical Ethics in the organization of medical service in a community." Doctors in Washington and Oregon had pioneered in county society plans as a defense against the industrial contract practice that proliferated in the region. The Pierce County Service Bureau of Washington formed in 1917, followed by other county bureaus. The King County Medical Service Bureau of Seattle formed in 1933 against the specific objections of *JAMA* editor Morris Fishbein. The bureaus established nonprofit corporations to act as agents in medical service contracts with employee and low-income groups. They differed from other forms of contract practice because they were professionally rather than lay directed, included all medical society members, and were strictly for medical service, not hospitalization. In 1939 the AMA sanctioned 150 of these plans in its publication *Organized Payment of Medical Services*, with the caveat that payment for "the individual, personal, scientific ministrations of the physician" remain "absolutely distinct from the payment for hospital care."[3]

In 1943 the AMA announced its intent to establish a nationwide association as a physician's corollary to the American Hospital Association's Blue Cross Commission. By 1946 forty-three state society plans had an enrollment of three million people. The following year Associated Medical Care was renamed the Blue Shield Commission. Doctors of Washington State medical societies again showed fierce independence, remaining independent of Blue Shield. In 1943 Blue Cross also began streamlining its hospital network, with policies such as reciprocal membership transfer among Blue Cross plans nationally and cooperation in enrolling national accounts such as those with the big labor unions.[4]

Analysts attribute the rapid development of Blue Cross and Blue Shield on the West Coast to geographic isolation, rapid and large-scale industrialization, and the resulting proliferation of prepaid group plans by employers and workers. Sociologist Paul Starr synthesizes the argument: "The response of the medical profession to Kaiser was entirely in keeping with the long-term pattern of defensive prepayment adopted ever since physicians in Washington and Oregon set up their own plans to fight commercial prepayment plans."[5]

Henry Kaiser stayed on the offensive against the societies. He met threats by the local ACMA-controlled Procurement and Assignment Service to draft his physicians by going directly to the national level and Boston-based chair of the service, Dr. Frank H. Lahey, then delegated negotiations to Garfield, who focused on the poor physical condition of both the huge labor force and Permanente physicians. He made the physicians sound decrepit. Two-thirds of them were army rejects or over thirty-seven years of age. Of the thirty-nine doctors at Richmond at the end of 1942, twelve were over forty years old, a couple of these nearing sixty-five. Fourteen had physical defects and were rejected by the military. Only thirteen were "healthy and active." It was the "healthy and active" third of the physician staff that Garfield fought to keep, prime candidates for the military draft in November 1942, at the start of peak build-up of shipyard production. Garfield wrote Lahey that all were "key men" without whom the group over thirty-seven years of age and those unfit for military service could not operate as a "competent medical service."[6]

Federal officials recognized that Kaiser was essential to the war effort and usually ruled in his favor in cases of key personnel and materials allotment. At times approval for Kaiser requests came from Franklin Roosevelt's office.[7]

Kaiser also triumphed in the public forum of the U.S. Senate. The Committee on Education and Labor chaired by outspoken liberal Florida senator Claude Pepper held hearings on the health care of civilian war workers in November 1942, shortly after the exchange with Fletcher and Garfield's plea to Lahey.

Pepper dramatized complaints by Kaiser and Garfield to the committee that the county societies prevented them from treating family members of Kaiser workers at Portland-Vancouver. The two men also complained of the threats by the local Procurement and Assignment committees to draft Kaiser Permanente physicians. Pepper expressed horror that U.S. citizens, civilian war producers, were deprived of adequate health care for their families because of medical society obstruction.

The senator challenged *JAMA* editor Morris Fishbein's professional credentials and his involvement with the procurement and draft boards. Fishbein then lambasted Kaiser, Garfield, and the Permanente medical staff. He declared to his colleagues nationwide that Kaiser's efforts to obtain restricted building material and equipment for his hospitals, and draft exemption for his physicians, represented "the desire of some industrial leaders and of their full-time staffs of physicians which they employ to maintain their individual empires without disturbance." Kaiser challenged Fishbein in subsequent U.S. Senate testimony. He referred to his work force as an "Army of Production" and characterized the Permanente outpatient treatment program that kept workers mobile as "an assembly line of men."[8]

The industrialist continued to expand his facilities. A third addition to the Oakland hospital was completed in February 1943, yet it remained "badly overcrowded." Henry Kaiser applied for funds and material allocations to increase the bed capacity from 135 to 250, and for an addition to the Richmond Field Hospital of 100 beds. In March 1943 Garfield wrote a personal note to Henry Kaiser that revealed his anxiety. Admitting that he had not slept well after a tense conversation with Kaiser, Garfield vowed to defer to Kaiser's judgment in carrying out expansion: "I want to let you know that I am convinced you were absolutely right and of course I was wrong in arguing with you. My eagerness to treat everybody and to amortize rapidly threw me off balance. As to the doctors you were again right. We should not be afraid of them—so please forget and forgive. I'll try not to trouble you again. I bow to your greater wisdom."[9] The simple note revealed the clear lines of authority and deference between the two men that characterized their relationship until Henry Kaiser's death.

The report of the East Bay Hospital Conference held by the

ACMA in June denied that a bed shortage existed in the area. The motive was clear. The report charged that neither local physicians nor hospitals wished to lose potential paying patients, or to see "further expansion of the corporate practice of medicine." Five months later, Procurement and Assignment chair Harold Fletcher triumphantly read a teletype from the War Production Board at the local meeting, denying priority for the Oakland Permanente Hospital addition because no bed shortage in the area existed. Garfield, who was present at the meeting, accused the Oakland physicians of "blocking the construction of our hospital." He insisted that a shortage existed and that the doctors present "know that in your own hearts." The Kaiser organization had enough beds for its workers, he went on, but was concerned about the families of employees. Permanente facilities opened to the public would provide a critical community service. Only two of the thirteen local doctors present supported Garfield's call for a new survey of bed space.[10]

The San Francisco Urgency Committee turned the tables on Kaiser's vaunted patriotism, charging that government support gave Kaiser "special privileges" and that federal funding of Kaiser projects was excessive. Facilities available to Kaiser workers were "luxurious" in contrast to the canvas tents for fighting men in the field. They implied that the $250,000 profit the Permanente Foundation reaped from the hospital enterprise was unconscionable. But local doctors had a pyrrhic victory. Kaiser again ignored local opinion. Praising Works Project Administration (WPA) vice-president Wilson for his foresighted recognition of the medical needs of war producers, the industrialist presented his own survey of medical needs in the East Bay. "We have always thought of ourselves," he wrote to Wilson, "in regard to this hospital activity, as being the only ones in the territory who had initiative enough to provide medical care for our shipyard workers." Just as Fishbein had warned, Kaiser's ambition stretched well beyond his own industry. "We would be very happy to provide medical care for all of the defense workers in the territory," he wrote, "just to prevent the costly absenteeism due to ill health."[11]

The national Urgency Committee overturned the local committee and approved 200 additional beds for Richmond and

Oakland at the beginning of 1944. In 1943 and 1944 Permanente Health Plan membership averaged 76,000 employees in northern California, with thousands more eligible when space was available. The federal government not only agreed that Kaiser medical facilities and personnel were essential to the war effort, it pumped in generous funds. The FWA granted $220,000 to Northern Permanente at Portland-Vancouver, developed the Richmond Field Hospital on a rental agreement with Permanente, and funded the 1944 addition to the Permanente Hospital in Oakland. Kaiser and Garfield came up with private funds of $800,000 for the Portland-Vancouver facilities and well over $600,000 in northern California.[12]

In 1943, the year of peak production in the Kaiser shipyards, AMA conservatives experienced other major setbacks. First in 1939, then from 1943 (as S. 1320) through the rest of the decade (as S. 1679 and H.R. 4312), New York senator Robert Wagner, along with Senator James Murray of Montana and Representative John Dingell of Michigan, introduced bills to add health insurance to the welfare programs under the Federal Security Agency. The Wagner bills kept organization on a traditional fee-for-service basis in what was primarily a payment plan, a far cry from socialized medicine.[13] Conservatives saw the 1943 version as more extreme than Wagner's 1939 proposal because it called for federal rather than state management of health and welfare services.[14]

The first Wagner-Murray-Dingell bill appeared the same year as the landmark Supreme Court decision against the AMA and District of Columbia medical society for "restraint of trade" against GHA of Washington, D.C. The antitrust suit brought by the Department of Justice was upheld in *AMA v. U.S.*[15] The GHA decision signified the beginning of a long slide in prestige and authority for the AMA and its membership of solo fee-for-service physicians. It deflated the mystical aura and elitism of U.S. medicine, bringing the health reform debate into the arena shared by other interest groups in U.S. society.[16]

Labor supported both Wagner and Kaiser. As union members rapidly enrolled in Permanente during 1945, the ILWU kept members informed about the status of Wagner-Murray-Dingell, an omnibus health bill by Florida Democrat Pepper, and state bills for prepaid compulsory health insurance. The union continued its vociferous opposition to the AMA. Its newspaper charged the AMA with "running a red, white and blue campaign for medical profits" and spending enough in one month on lobbying and advertising to provide complete health care to every ILWU member and their families for two years. Union journalists treated the AMA as a common corporate monopoly: "As a trade union concerned with the welfare of . . . all American workers, we condemn this conspicuous waste [by the AMA] . . . by distorting the truth to preserve its monopoly and the drug monopoly," and the union vowed "to resist and expose this big business combine against the nation's health."[17]

The Sacramento statehouse also threatened California doctors. Between 1941 and 1945, eighty-two compulsory insurance bills appeared in thirteen states. In California five appeared between 1935 and 1949. Governor Earl Warren's administration supported a steady stream of proposals for state insurance that echoed the series introduced in U.S. congressional committees. The two public insurance movements, and opposition against them, ran parallel through the rest of the decade. Yet the Warren bills called for less inclusive benefits than those offered by CPS in 1939, and both limited coverage to those with incomes under $3,000.[18] By the time Warren went to the Supreme Court in 1953, no state insurance legislation had been enacted.

In deference to Permanente physicians who wanted a low public profile, Kaiser officials sought to minimize identification with the governor's controversial views, though Warren represented the progressive California political environment that countered medical society opposition to Kaiser.[19]

The CMA hired the San Francisco public relations firm of Whitaker and Baxter for $100,000 a year to advertise against Warren's health insurance plan. The AMA was also a Whitaker and Baxter client, using the incendiary rhetoric of international conflict to turn public opinion against the welfare state as a form of German, then Soviet, totalitarianism. The AMA spent $129,000, from November 1942 through October 1943, in the antiinsurance campaign, and over $2 million a year by the end of the decade, obtained by assessing individual members.[20]

Whitaker and Baxter distributed fifty-five million copies of a pamphlet for the AMA entitled "The Voluntary Way is the American Way," the campaign motto. "Why is compulsory insurance called socialized medicine?" it queried the public. Government control meant "control not only of the medical profession, but of hospitals—both public and private—the drug and appliance industries, dentistry, pharmacy, nursing and allied professions." Government would "dominate the medical affairs of every citizen," with central administrative lines extending from Washington, D.C., "down through state, town, district, and neighborhood bureaus." Lenin had declared "socialized medicine . . . the keystone to the arch of the socialist state." Senator Murray researched the Lenin quote and could find no such statement in his speeches or writings.[21] Historical verification was not covered in the AMA's $1.5 million budget.

AMA dogmas of individualism and the sanctity of the personal doctor-patient trust ran counter to realities recognized by the U.S. public. Popular periodicals emphasizing the idea of limitless medical progress, scientific breakthroughs during the war, and the nationalist spirit accustomed Americans to see good medical care as an inalienable right. The public demanded affordable access to the best science had to offer. A *Fortune* poll in 1942 indicated that 74 percent of those interviewed favored national health insurance; a Gallup poll in 1943 put the level at 59 percent. A 1943 *JAMA* survey indicated majority support of insurance among military physicians (half of all physicians under age 65) planning to enter private practice after the war. Another poll result may have encouraged conservative acceptance of private plans like Kaiser Permanente as a lesser evil than state or national medicine; only about a third of the population surveyed preferred national health insurance to private prepaid plans offered through place of employment if given the latter option.[22]

The positive attitude toward group prepayment indicated what one historian calls "a revolution" in health care financing without government involvement. In June 1943 the AMA study found that more than 1.5 million employees and dependents were enrolled in 124 industrial prepayment plans. Also, twenty-three private group practice plans with prepayment had enrolled almost 400,000 subscribers, and thirty consumer-sponsored prepayment plans had over 185,000 members. Yet these numbers were minuscule at a time when total union membership was 13.6 million, and the U.S. population was 136.7 million.[23]

Private insurance covered the larger number of Americans, with Blue Cross hospitalization plans the most common form of insurance. Only 9 percent of hospital patients had insurance in 1940, but by 1951, more than half were insured, with Blue Shield membership at 37.4 million. Also, by 1951, more than 40 million people had private insurance to pay physicians' bills, the vast majority by indemnity payments to patients who would then personally reimburse their doctors.[24] Blue Cross and Blue Shield thus sustained the traditional individualized structure of health care.

The year following the GHA victory in court, the AMA withdrew its opposition to the popular wartime hero, Henry Kaiser, leaving the field to its local affiliates. With the renewed threat of national insurance, the legal setback in the GHA case, and public disapproval of its expensive lobbying effort against the insurance bills, the association needed allies, not enemies. Moreover, Kaiser and *JAMA* editor Morris Fishbein both opposed government insurance.

Public relations triumphs through 1944 put Kaiser and Garfield in the national reform spotlight, as New York mayor Fiorello La Guardia appointed a committee to formulate a medical insurance program, incorporated in 1944 as the Health Insurance Plan of Greater New York, and New York philanthropist Mary Lasker persuaded Kaiser to be a HIP incorporator.[25] Less than a month after Kaiser agreed to support HIP, Garfield made a triumphant visit to the East Coast as Lasker's guest in order to advise the New Yorkers. The New Yorkers felt they must provide a choice in order to gain the support of organized medicine, or at least not provoke its opposition. But Garfield told them that HIP would not succeed if operated on a combination closed and open panel basis, that is, if some doctors worked exclusively for HIP and others maintained independent practices. He noted other "stumbling blocks" were "medical politics" in the East, the fact that facilities were owned by outside interests, and the involvement in Blue Cross. Garfield also dined and conferred with the elite of East Coast academic medicine, the directors of New York University and Columbia University medical schools; with HIP founder and director of Mt. Sinai Hospital Dr. George Baehr; and with La Guardia himself. Garfield wrote to Kaiser that he had a pleasant dinner with Morris Fishbein, who took credit for Garfield's invitation to speak before the AMA Congress on Industrial Health at which Garfield outlined the principles of health maintenance.[26]

In January 1945 *Fortune* magazine published companion letters by La Guardia and Garfield that illustrated the difference between HIP and the Kaiser plan. HIP combined prepayment and numerous independent practice groups scattered throughout the service area. Kaiser Permanente fully integrated prepayment with full-time Permanente medical groups and facilities. Garfield stressed that facilities were essential to success, yet beyond the means of other plans to provide because of cost and the obstructive power of local medical interests.[27]

Despite these forays among Eastern reformers and liberal politicians, Henry Kaiser disappointed those who directly sought his aid. Kaiser wrote Mary Lasker, who solicited his support for Wagner-Murray-Dingell in 1943, that the bill was "too comprehensive." Senator Wagner also asked for the industrialist's support, requesting his advice for changes in the bill. He responded to Wagner in terms of traditional Republican values, expressing his belief in voluntarism, private enterprise, individual responsibility, and the work ethic. He was convinced, he told Wagner, that it was the responsibility of employers, working with physicians, to provide health plans and facilities for their workers, countering the tendency toward socialized medicine as manifest in postwar European nations. Kaiser's attorneys objected to his involvement with the liberal East Coast politicians and extricated him from identification with HIP. He declined La Guardia's invitation to join the HIP board of directors in January 1945 with the excuse that he had to devote all energies to the war effort.[28]

Privately Kaiser and Garfield decided that the Wagner bill was not in their best interest. Garfield thought that it would result in a "general deterioration" of medical care. In his 1944 remarks before the AMA, he stated that the Kaiser plan "would protect against the 'Federalization of Medicine'," that "the members of our plan receive more medical care than the Wagner Act would provide," and that the government would not attempt to "federalize" medicine "if the need was non-existent." He emphasized that the Kaiser plan was one "operated by the physicians themselves."[29] West Coast doctors did not believe the Permanente doctors had autonomy from the corporate board room. They maintained objection to lay control of medical practice, whether from government or corporate interests.

Yet on the national stage Kaiser appealed to a broad range of politicians from Wagner to Taft. In March 1945 he produced a detailed proposal for national expansion of the Permanente model. He advocated a national system of prepayment through place of employment to medical care organizations operated in conjunction with a physician's group such as Sidney R. Garfield and Associates. These organizations would operate in facilities financed by a federal health and housing agency such as the Federal Housing Administration (FHA). The government agency would grant loans for up to 90 percent of construction costs, amortized over twenty years. The proposed system would serve 100 million people and would cost each individual member only fifty-eight cents a week, Kaiser figured. It would employ another 1.8 million health care workers and professionals. If operated as efficiently as the Kaiser Permanente program, the national plan would cost workers less than 4 percent of their yearly wages.[30]

Membership in the country's prepaid group plans was small in the mid-1940s and drew from certain occupational categories. Also, members tended to appear left of center in postwar politics. In 1946, the first year Kaiser was offered to the public, prominent proponents included New Deal–era federal and state bureaucrats of GHA; the Health Service System, begun in 1938 in California; GHA of Washington, D.C.; and the Health Insurance Plan (HIP) of New York. At that time, also, more than 85 percent of UMW members, well over 52,000 miners nationally, were members of prepaid plans (see table 3.1).[31] Aggressive unionists, government employees, and liberal academic institutions led the Kaiser membership explosion between 1945 and 1955.

National planning was a common subject of political discourse in the immediate postwar period, and not unique to

TABLE 3.1. Selected Prepaid Group Health Plans, 1955

Year Founded	Prepaid Group Plan	Sponsorship	Members
1929	Farmer's Union Hospital Association, Elk City, Oklahoma	Consumer	7,200
1929	Ross-Loos Medical Group, Los Angeles	Private group practice	139,622
1937	Group Health Association, Inc., Washington, D.C. (GHA)	Consumer	20,214
1942	Kaiser Foundation Health Plan, California	Kaiser shipbuilding	450,297[a]
1945	Health Insurance Plan of Greater New York (HIP)	Consumer	415,152
1946	United Mine Workers Welfare and Retirement Funds	Employer-union	1,000,000

SOURCE: AMA, Report of the Commission on Medical Care Plans, part 2, appendix C (AMA: May 1958; rev. October 1958), *JAMA Special Edition* (17 January 1959), 24–36.
[a]Kaiser records 478,000 at the end of 1954. The AMA survey notes that it did not know of Northwest Permanente at the time.

Kaiser. Ideas connecting health and broad social planning were rapidly implemented by European policymakers but defeated in the United States. Though based on capitalist rather than socialist economics, important Kaiser Permanente objectives corresponded more closely to those of the British National Health Service (NHS) established in 1946 than to the atomistic, science-based U.S. system. Like Kaiser, the British focused on working-class access. Health was an organic component of community planning, and both areas were placed within the Ministry of Health. The Kaiser blueprint for maintaining health was designed for a productive citizenry, not as an asylum for the permanently dependent. Henry Kaiser would concur with the Fabian socialists who supported the

British Compulsory Insurance Act in 1911 and the Beveridge Report in 1942. They stressed the "personal responsibility" of workers to comply with the national health care goals to counter the "waste and expense of disease." Here similarities with Kaiser's views ceased. The British system sought to "absorb" or "replace" all existing public services and to integrate voluntary hospitals.[32]

Competition and consumer choice among a variety of plans were essential to Kaiser's plan. Free choice assured quality, economy, and mutual commitment by the patient and doctor to the patient's health. The principle of competition on the free market eliminated the passive dependency of the patient and guarded against bureaucratic inertia within the doctors' groups. Kaiser's plan was thoroughly grounded in principles of economic liberalism. Government should provide "easily available funds through a loaning agency for facilities," Garfield wrote to the secretary of commerce, Henry A. Wallace, and let the "free-swinging, competitive type of American enterprise enter the field of prepayment and group practice in adequate facilities." It was his "sincere conviction" that "this country would see the most brilliant advance in quality and spread of medical care ever witnessed."[33]

Kaiser's views were endorsed by liberal senators Lister Hill, James Murray, and Claude Pepper, who were "especially impressed" by his "National Health Plan." It was the best "method for stabilizing and rationalizing the economics of medical practice," he told Pepper, "within the system of free private enterprise." Because it was so firmly grounded in consensus politics, Kaiser believed his plan "should meet no objection from the medical profession and should invite the support of all groups who are concerned by the problem of extending complete prepaid medical service to the people."[34]

Nevertheless, the entrepreneurial group practitioner described by Garfield was decades away from acceptance by the medical profession. In 1940 group physicians represented only 1.2 percent of the profession; by 1946 only 2.6 percent of U.S. doctors practiced in groups. AMA conservatives continued to view group practice as socialistic if income was pooled and then redistributed among group practitioners.[35]

Health care issues faded in the public forum as rapid demobilization rekindled labor-capital disputes over wages. In September 1945 the United Steelworkers of America and the UAW demanded a 30 percent wage increase to offset the 22.3 percent rise in consumer prices. With union membership at nearly fourteen million, over 20 percent of the steelworkers and more than 50 percent of the automobile workers went on strike.[36]

In the midst of the labor crisis in November 1945 Harry Truman became the first president to recommend a comprehensive national health program to Congress. He gave an address entirely devoted to a redraft of Wagner-Murray-Dingell. In the spring of 1946 almost a million rail and coal workers went on strike. The federal government seized the railroads and mines, and the White House helped miners' and steelworkers' unions gain an 18.5 cent-an-hour pay raise. While other capitalists refused Truman's wage hike, Kaiser signed the agreement during the steel strike with CIO president Philip Murray at the White House. As labor battles raged at General Motors, Kaiser kept peace at his Willow Run plant near Detroit at Ypsilanti. Michigan law and the "active antagonism generated by the local medical profession" made it impossible for the company to form a Kaiser Health Plan. But the union administrator of the Kaiser-Frazer health and welfare program reported that Kaiser was first in the industry to establish a company-paid hospital and surgical coverage plan through Blue Cross and Blue Shield. He also was next after Ford with a company paid pension.[37]

In the 1946 National Bituminous Coal Mine Wage, or Krugs-Lewis, Agreement, the UMW won unprecedented "fringe benefits" that included vacation pay, a guaranteed work week with overtime pay, a revised Federal Mine Safety Code, and a welfare and retirement fund paid by the mine operators through a five cent-a-ton royalty charge. Nevertheless UMW and CIO leader John L. Lewis accused the Truman White House of reneging and threatened another strike. Truman turned on Lewis and other left-wing labor leaders, singling out two powerful Kaiser Permanente advocates. In the draft of a speech before Congress on the railroad strike, the

President referred to CIO leader Philip Murray and "his Communist friends." He called for his "comrades in arms" to "eliminate the Lewises" and "the Communist Bridges," Harry Bridges of the ILWU. Aides deleted most of the inflammatory remarks before the address.[38] Truman had singled out two of the staunchest supporters of prepaid group health in the labor movement, and both had close connections with Kaiser's health plan.

Like Bridges, Lewis presided over a membership whose solidarity and militancy stemmed from their work in a rugged natural resource industry. Yet Lewis had a much larger, multi-regional constituency in an essential national industry. UMW members numbered 416,000 by 1950 and mined 90 percent of the nation's coal.[39] Aggressive unionists like Lewis and Bridges supported Kaiser's brand of welfare capitalism because the unions had neither the economic power to build a labor health system, or the political strength to effect state or federal health insurance legislation.

West Coast labor leaders recognized the obstacles to union health centers. Most of an estimated twenty-five centers sponsored by seven unions in the 1950s were east of the Mississippi River and limited to diagnosis and outpatient treatment for workers only.[40] The AMA county affiliates followed a now-familiar pattern of obstruction. They blocked labor center doctors from membership and denied them hospital privileges. Neither unions nor contract physicians had adequate financial resources to establish their own comprehensive facilities.

By 1952 union members and their families represented over half the population of San Francisco. AFL locals comprised 90 percent of the 225,000 union members in the city.[41] Both the CIO-ILWU and the AFL San Francisco Labor Council faltered in brief health center movements in the early 1950s. Both used a Yale University public health expert, Dr. E. Richard Weinerman, as chief consultant, who first came west to work with Garfield in 1951. Weinerman's studies revealed the complex financial and professional barriers to union plans.[42] Kaiser Permanente thus remained an acceptable alternative for California union leaders, who also continued to lobby for state insurance. Kaiser continued to use the health plan as a broad avenue of communication with them.

The Steelworkers and United Auto Workers pioneered in nationwide insurance programs for their members with Blue Cross and Blue Shield. UAW president Walter Reuther's continued bargaining efforts and a National Labor Relations Board ruling in 1949 enabled the extension of the Permanente Health Plan to the UAW in California in the early 1950s. The NLRB ruled that General Motors (GM) was committing an unfair labor practice by refusing to bargain for health benefits. In 1950 the company agreed to pay half of hospital and surgical coverage for workers and their dependents. Ford and Chrysler soon followed, and over one million UAW members and families came under similar health coverage agreements. Reuther was dissatisfied with the limited Blue Cross–Blue Shield coverage, which did not provide preventive and outpatient care. Along with UAW social security director Harry Becker, he extolled the comprehensive programs of HIP on the East Coast and Kaiser Permanente in the West.[43]

There were 31,500 UAW workers at GM, Chevrolet, Buick, International Harvester, Ford, Lincoln-Mercury, Studebaker, and a variety of other companies up and down the California coast. Garfield now sought to force Blue Cross–Blue Shield acceptance of a "free choice" principle in their contracts with the unions by educating Reuther and Kaiser's wartime ally, GM president Charles E. Wilson, about the Kaiser economic advantages. In order to compete with the advertised subscription rates of Blue Cross–Blue Shield, Kaiser lowered rates in 1946 to $5.25 for a subscriber with two or more dependents, from a high of $8.45 in 1946. To offset the additional expenses for Kaiser's comprehensive care, the administration levied minimal office visit fees of $1 and $2 for house calls. But this was not the main reason that Kaiser could compete financially with the other plans. Kaiser administrative costs at 9 percent were half that of the 18 percent spent by Blue Cross. Kaiser and Garfield succeeded in establishing the "free choice" principle and gained thousands of UAW members in California.[44]

In 1953 and 1954 Ford auto workers in Richmond, and the Steelworkers in South San Francisco and Pittsburg, assumed Kaiser coverage as a local supplement to a national Blue Cross plan. The workers paid the supplement, though U.S. Steel agreed to payroll deductions for this purpose.[45]

Aggressive labor leaders had pushed liberal government to its farthest reaches in U.S. welfare politics. Conservatives attacked the labor movement for its decade and a half of militancy that began on the West Coast in 1934 with the waterfront strike led by Harry Bridges's longshoremen. Republican senator Robert Taft led the backlash that surfaced in 1946, with support first of the Case bill, then of the Taft-Hartley bill. Punitive measures in the bills included the prohibition of health and welfare funds paid by employers but administered by unions, and of group insurance and hospitalization as the subjects of collective bargaining. Liberals barely sustained Truman's veto of the Case bill; Taft-Hartley was passed over his veto. Fortunately for welfare unionists the antihealth and antiwelfare elements were deleted before final action. Subsequent agreements and a court ruling affirmed union direction over benefits. Nevertheless, after the November 1945 health message, Truman withdrew from the health care battleground.[46]

Now Wagner-Murray-Dingell infuriated conservatives and did not have moderate support. Kaiser lobbyists pushed for a hospital financing bill introduced by Lyndon B. Johnson that authorized the Reconstruction Finance Corporation to make 40 percent grants for facilities construction. Kaiser's comment to Lasker that the Wagner bill was "too comprehensive" was a euphemism for less conciliatory descriptions. On the first day of hearings on the bill in April 1946, committee chair James Murray requested witnesses to refrain from characterizing it as "communistic" or "socialistic." Archconservative senator Robert Taft retorted that he considered it "socialism . . . the most socialistic measure that this Congress has ever had before it." Murray refused Taft further recognition. The Ohio senator abruptly left the hearing room and did not attend further sessions. A parade of opposition witnesses included the American Hospital Association, Blue Cross, the American

Bar Association, the U.S. Chamber of Commerce, and the National Grange.[47]

Yet the liberal thrust produced a moderate-conservative compromise to provide federal funding for hospitals under state and local AMA control. After his fellow Ohio senator Harold Burton went to the Supreme Court, Taft became Senate sponsor of the Hill-Burton Hospital Survey and Construction bill, signed into law by Truman on 13 August 1946. A 1940 bill had called for direct federal financing and ownership of hospitals. Hill-Burton initiated a program of federal grants to the states for survey and construction, with control at the local level. Hill-Burton administrators would not enter the doctor's realm of medical service.

The emphasis on facilities and scientific education epitomized health policy of the 1940s, according to social welfare historian Edward Berkowitz, the pragmatic legacies of the CCMC and Blue Cross in the preceding decade. The surgeon general, Dr. Thomas Parran, stated the appeal of the measure: it supported "expansion in the name of hospital science," and the idea of the modern hospital as "a complex technical machine."[48]

Hill-Burton was at odds with the egalitarian and preventive medicine principles supported by labor and liberal reformers. There was no formula for equitable access or for the formation of group practices to staff the burgeoning institutional system, which by 1952 included 80,000 new beds supplied at a cost of $1.4 billion.[49] Moreover, neither Hill-Burton nor the Veterans Administration Act required racial integration of federally supported facilities. It was hardly "the purest form of democracy," as it was melodramatically labeled by the AMA speaker at the Hill-Burton congressional hearings.[50]

Kaiser trustees did not voice formal opposition to Hill-Burton but realized it would be of no benefit to their program because AMA opponents would not admit the need for more hospital beds in the regions served by Kaiser Permanente. Kaiser successfully appealed to congressional conservatives in discussion of the measure, however. In a telephone conversation with Kaiser on modifications of Hill-Burton, Taft said that he was "very much taken" with Kaiser's program for U.S.

workers, though he was "afraid we can't write the bill for that alone. . . . We have to make *some* grants for the indigent."[51] Henry Kaiser subscribed to the old bootstrap progressivism of Theodore Roosevelt rather than to the welfare state of New Deal and Fair Deal Democrats.

Meanwhile, animosities again flared in the West Coast county medical societies against Permanente physician leaders. Ernest Saward and seven physicians who remained with him at war's end at Portland and Vancouver announced intentions to continue the program after the shipyards closed. Saward was the only Permanente doctor with membership in the Clark County Medical Society. The Washington State Medical Society notified him that it "disapproved" of Northern Permanente's "mode of operation" and that doctors associated with it were "unethical." Meetings between Saward and state society representatives failed to resolve problems, and Saward appealed the ethics allegation to the AMA Judicial Council in December 1945.

In June 1946 the council withdrew the formal charge of "unethical practice" against Northern Permanente. But stresses remained. Within a year, first medical director Wallace Neighbor, who had begun with Garfield at Grand Coulee, left for Oakland. He fled more than the enmity of his medical society colleagues. Large financial problems, the difficult veteran patient population, and the apparent political radicalism of other doctors in the program combined to give him angina attacks. Saward thought they were psychosomatic. "Wally wanted out," he said. "He really didn't want to be involved in anything as abrasive and controversial as what we were going through." Problems included internal politics. There were radicals among the handful of doctors who remained after the war. Saward described one as "quite liberal" and "eccentric." Two others, he said, "were *very* far to the left—people who were to some extent hounded by the FBI" and "joined all the causes of the day." They were "clearly way to the left of the center of American public opinion." In fact, he later concluded, they were "doctrinaire Marxists." Until they were "forced out" by unspecified circumstances in 1950, Saward admitted, their ideological commitment was important as Northern Permanente membership shrank to 3,000. But the "left-leaning activity" of the group eventually "cast a shadow" on the program. Even the liberal Saward had trouble tolerating the "dialectic struggle" with them and saw that they were "a great detriment in community relations" as reactionary Cold War rhetoric began to dominate domestic political debate.[52]

Sidney Garfield faced more severe problems with the California medical establishment. While national AMA leaders mollified Kaiser and channeled energies into the larger fight against liberal Democrats in Congress, the county societies in the San Francisco Bay Area launched a direct assault on Garfield. The California State Board of Medical Examiners and the Ethics Committee of the Alameda County Medical Association charged Garfield with violation of the state Medical Practice Act on 23 May 1946. After a hearing in San Francisco, the case was continued to the following summer.[53]

In 1945 and 1946 Garfield employed several doctors as interns or residents who did not have California licenses. The major complaint was against the employment of Dr. Clifford Keene, later president of Kaiser Permanente. Keene's professional credentials were sound; he was a board-certified surgeon from Michigan who had directed major military medical facilities during the war. But he was not a legal resident of California. Garfield also was accused of keeping seven other interns on staff who were not licensed in the state and of employing until 1946 a physician who had had his license revoked for drug use. The medical board placed Garfield on five years' probation and suspended his license for one year. He appealed on the grounds that eight of the physicians were in training and not required to have licenses. The case of the ninth physician was under appeal, and the state attorney general had ruled it legal to keep him on the payroll until his case was decided.[54]

Garfield avoided further controversy. One month after the board passed sentence he refused to join in an antitrust investigation of the AMA by a Minnesota law firm representing the Cooperative Health Federation of America. Pioneering creator of the prepaid group plan in Elk City, Oklahoma, Dr. Michael Shadid, was a prominent participant. The firm sought investigation of "restraint of trade" violations by medical societies nationwide through the U.S. attorney general. An investigation into lobbying by large special interests carried out by the Justice Department included fifteen state and county medical societies for actions against the plans. The AMA reacted by charging the Truman administration with "police tactics."[55]

Garfield declined the invitation to submit evidence of discrimination against Permanente doctors. He indicated a firm resolve to keep a low profile in regard to the AMA in his two-sentence response to the lawyers: "This organization has not experienced discriminatory action of sufficient importance to warrant any charges against the Medical Association. In fact many of the physicians in the American Medical Association have assisted us a great deal in accomplishing our work."[56]

Others were more aggressive in Garfield's defense. In September 1947 ILWU officials were talking with Permanente administrators about coastwide enrollment of its membership in the Permanente Health Plan, and encouraging expansion in southern California. The ILWU *Dispatcher* reported on 22 October that suspension of Garfield's license had begun the "long-awaited all-out campaign to drive the Permanente Foundation Hospital here out of business."[57]

Henry Kaiser loudly protested general press coverage of *Garfield v. the Board of Medical Examiners*. He wrote to six Bay Area newspapers calling the allegations against his physician chief "obscure technical violations of the medical licensing regulation." Overwrought, Kaiser became melodramatic, using biblical analogies. False accusations by a loud minority who wanted to destroy the health plan were outweighed by the belief of "the many who would not wish this physician to suffer." They could say, intoned Kaiser, as did Pontius Pilate, "'I can see no wrong in this man, but let us turn him over to the State.' For myself, I know this man's life is being spent in serving others." He emphasized the physician's "personal sacrifices," concluding, "Of those who would do him evil in their efforts to destroy our plan of medical care, I can only say, 'God forgive them for they know not what they do'."[58]

On 8 June 1948 the ACMA served notice that its council

was proceeding with the charges of unprofessional conduct against Garfield first leveled eight months before. A hearing was set for 16 September. Kaiser met with Bay Area doctors on 9 June in what he euphemistically called an "off the record discussion of mutual problems." He was "profoundly shocked," and indeed "astounded and horrified," when his attorneys had informed him that afternoon that Alameda County doctors "have declared war on the Permanente health program." Kaiser shared personal vignettes to gain sympathy from his audience. He also appealed to the doctors' self-interest. His medical program would counter the need, he claimed, for "the otherwise inevitable future imposition of Government medicine." Abruptly shifting from a supplicating tone to one of chastisement, Kaiser scolded them for their selfish conduct.[59]

The ACMA charges were more extreme than the state board case, extending well beyond the charge of employing unlicensed doctors. They were a catalog of the same objections to corporate-sponsored prepaid group plans articulated by the AMA since the 1930s. Garfield was charged with "advertising and solicitation of patients," placing "mass production ahead of the health needs of the patients," denial of "free choice of physicians, false promises of medical care to thousands of patients who, because of inadequate staffing, received poor quality service," and "profit" from Garfield and Associates.

Kaiser warned that the Permanente trustees would not tolerate continued attacks on the integrity of the medical program and its doctors. His attorneys already had sufficient evidence for litigation, Kaiser threatened, against the Alameda and San Francisco county medical societies under federal antitrust statues. He urged them to "recall" the conviction of the AMA and District of Columbia society "for a similar attack upon a prepaid group plan." "If as we believe," he stated, "a conspiracy to restrain the practice of medicine exists, the state of California is by law obligated to proceed with dissolution of the medical associations." "This," concluded Kaiser, "is the end of the recommendations from our attorneys." He still preferred "a spirit of peace" to war and hoped the good doctors would join him in implementing his "solution" to the national health care problem.[60]

Five months later, in November 1948, Truman's surprise reelection would prove to be the last victory of the New Deal liberal coalition. Regular Democrats barely blocked challenges from the Progressive party splinter led by Henry Wallace. For the last time in more than a decade to come, they defeated conservative Republicans. Truman had just managed to sustain New Deal social legislation with the modifications of the extreme provisions of Taft-Hartley. Now the right-wing backlash against liberal Democrats escalated, as evidenced by the Employees' Loyalty Program under the FBI and the National Security Act of 1947 establishing the CIA and military unification. After 1948 an anticommunist consensus permeated national politics. Conservative Republicans and the medical lobby warned persistently of the socialist implications of the welfare state sought by New Deal and Fair Deal Democrats. As a client of Whitaker and Baxter, the CMA continued to lobby against the succession of health insurance bills at the state level.[61]

In November 1949, however, during the last frenzied phase of the national AMA campaign against compulsory insurance, the ACMA withdrew the charges against Garfield. In 1950 a judge finally ruled that Keene was not a legal resident of the state at the time of his employment and therefore Dr. Garfield had violated the Medical Practice Act. Although the case was not finally disposed until May 1951, Keene was fully licensed, Garfield's year of probation had ended, and the case was moot.[62]

Nevertheless, the dispute had a lasting effect on the Kaiser Permanente corporate structure. Creation of the Northern California Permanente Medical Group and incorporation of Permanente Hospitals occurred in February 1948. The medical group was a partnership of seven physicians, including Garfield. As the dispute with the AMA societies in the Bay Area intensified, Garfield officially withdrew as a partner in July 1949 to defuse opposition. The partnership was reformed with eight founding partners who continued to act as the executive committee of the group until 1957. Chief of staff Cecil Cutting; the medical director at Oakland, John Paul Fitzgibbon; Wallace Neighbor, former director of Northern Permanente; chief of surgery LaMonte Baritell; chief of obstetrics/gynecology Robert King; and Morris Collen, Oakland medical chief were in this group.[63]

Also in 1948, Saward and the doctors in Portland reorganized themselves as a partnership in order to dispel the notion that they were salaried employees of Henry Kaiser. Saward became director of the health plan, the hospital, and the medical group. The Permanente Clinic was created to contract with the Kaiser Permanente Foundation to provide medical services, with doctors receiving a percentage of health plan dues. The first Northern Permanente board meeting was called in April 1946 to consider the percentage proposal. Saward claimed that the board was identical to that dominated by Kaiser and Garfield in Oakland and considered the proposal "apostasy." But Alonzo Ordway and attorney Tom McCarthy engineered a favorable vote, giving the northern doctors what they wanted—43 percent of health plan dues to operate all outpatient facilities and hospital medical services. According to Saward, the agreement so alienated Garfield that he *"never* came back" to Oregon.[64]

Henry Kaiser's attention stayed fixed on national politics. Apart from his passionate defense of Garfield, he stayed aloof from local medical squabbles through the decade. Ironically, the case against Garfield ended at the same time that Morris Fishbein was ousted as *JAMA* editor. Except for oblique attacks after the wartime Pepper hearings, Fishbein remained neutral toward Kaiser. He and his fellow physicians had more serious woes—declining public esteem as well as the perennial state and federal insurance bills.

Ignoring a crisis brewing in California among the Permanente physicians, Henry Kaiser entered what would be the final stage in his involvement with national health politics, seeking to maintain a centrist ground among vying interests in the health reform arena. As had World War II, the Korean conflict brought Kaiser before federal officials, pleading the "essentiality" of Permanente doctors on the home front. But there were new players on the national stage. Joseph P.

McCarthy first gained national attention on 9 February 1950 in a speech before the Republican Women's Club in Wheeling, West Virginia, when he claimed to hold in his hand a list of Communists in the U.S. State Department. For more than two years McCarthy intimidated liberals in both parties with a rapid fire of unsubstantiated charges. The AMA and its local affiliates became increasingly adept at using the anticommunist reactionary rhetoric in its battle against "socialized medicine" and prepaid group health.

The Korean crisis opened up special avenues of harassment against Permanente physicians by local medical leaders. As he had during World War II, Kaiser went straight to the top of the U.S. defense establishment in late 1951. He appealed directly on personal stationery to the directors of the National Production Authority, Federal Security Agency, and Office of Defense Mobilization, again with Charles E. Wilson. In less than two months Wilson granted Kaiser priority status for expansion of the San Francisco Permanente Hospital and exemption of his doctors from the military draft.[65] From 1940 to 1950, the national supply of new physicians fell from 10 to 30 percent behind demand for staffing hospital facilities, increased by Hill-Burton. The AMA had compromised on hospital construction but remained in firm control of professional education. Now the military wanted more of the scarce graduates. The doctors' draft law passed in 1950 was extended twice until it was allowed to expire in 1957. Physicians were eligible up to age fifty. In 1952, Sidney Garfield was forty-six, Cecil Cutting was forty-one, and other Permanente doctors were much younger.[66]

Dr. William L. Bender, chair of the Northern California Medical Association Advisory Committee to Selective Service, was antagonistic. In reply to the contention that key Permanente doctors were "essential," he remarked sarcastically that "no doctor could be considered indispensable," as Kaiser claimed, "for he might die."[67] The Kaiser staff carefully itemized Permanente's civil service to the nation. The organization provided medical care to 95,000 employees and dependents under health plan contracts at military installations and industries in the early 1950s. Strong parallels with the

World War II defense community were evident. There were almost 11,000 members still at Mare Island Naval Shipyard, over 5,000 at the San Francisco Naval Shipyard at Hunter's Point, and over 4,000 at Alameda Naval Air Station. Over 20,000 more members of the ILWU were employees of private shipyards and Pacific docks considered vital to defense; over 3,000 were workers in the steel industry and other industries dependent on steel. Research groups in plastics, oil, and fuel, such as Western Regional Laboratory and Shell Development, were represented also in the huge Bay Area membership, as were employees of Kaiser industries in aircraft, aluminum, construction, chemicals, electronics, magnesium, mining, refractors, and steel.[68]

The Kaiser defense network stretched far to the north and south. In the state of Washington, employees of the Hanford atomic project were served by Northern Permanente, while the Fontana Community Hospital served Fontana iron and steel plant employees. According to publicists, the medical program aided national defense workers and prevented strikes. As far inland as Dragarton, Utah, Kaiser staffed a hospital for UMW members employed by U.S. Steel. Inadequate health care threatened steel production on the West Coast when Dragarton workers went on strike. The Permanente service brought the miners back to the production line. Despite all of this public service, the hostile local draft boards, controlled by AMA doctors, threatened to draft thirteen Permanente physicians.

Kaiser himself manned the first line of defense against the physician draft. Garfield's case became top priority when he was reclassified 1-A and notified for his physical examination. Garfield and Kaiser appealed personally to the county medical association advisory board. The industrialist also took the lead in the cases of Drs. Morris Collen, Cecil Cutting, and young Frederick A. Pellegrin, who suddenly emerged as a Kaiser favorite. He was head of endocrinology and metabolic diseases at Kaiser's new hospital at Walnut Creek, near his own residence. Kaiser battled the draft board through 1953, schooling the navy on its dependence on the Kaiser Health Plan in the region.[69]

Garfield was not assured of exemption until early 1955 by the army surgeon general, who quipped in correspondence, "Wouldn't the AMA love to get Sid in the Army?" Kaiser appealed personally to selective service chief Hershey, who promised to aid the industrialist in his battle against the local draft board on behalf of the Permanente doctors. Kaiser presented the case to the president's National Selective Service Appeal Board, complete with membership charts showing a twelvefold increase in plan membership to 511,000 since 1946 and poster-sized photographs of new facilities in areas with large defense worker populations.[70] Kaiser fought the draft as part of a larger power struggle with the AMA. He was out to prove a point: his medical program had national significance superseding even that of the military medical establishment. Exemption of Permanente doctor administrators would be recognition of this at the highest level of government, recognition the local AMA doctors would abhor. Political stakes were high on both sides.

Despite Kaiser's stubbornness the Pellegrin case droned on. In 1956 Dr. Bender's local committee voted a last time against Pellegrin's essentiality. The board was hostile. One member asked Pellegrin how long it would take to find a replacement for him, adding, "No one is indispensable. What if you died? . . . Who would take your place if you took a two-year vacation?" "You will have to hurry up," another chimed in. "We have been gracious in granting you more time. But we cannot allow you further stalling. . . . This is getting monotonous your coming before us. Do you realize you would have twenty more years to come before us every six months for deferment?"[71]

Kaiser set an appeal in motion from Honolulu delaying Pellegrin's fate for eight more months, but ultimately the doctor was called up. He wrote Kaiser an emotional letter that expressed gratitude for the opportunity of working for him and "warm feelings of affection" for Kaiser and his wife. Kaiser promised to offer him an executive position with the medical program Kaiser planned for Hawaii. For the time being, though, the doctor faced a two-year stretch in the navy.[72]

In the interim, the political tide seemed to run in favor of the AMA. The election of Dwight D. Eisenhower in 1952 ended the twenty-year occupation of the White House by lib-

eral Democrats. AMA president Louis Bauer assured members, after the six million–vote Republican victory over Adlai
Stevenson, that "as far as the medical profession is concerned
. . . we are in less danger of socialization than for a number of
years." The new U.S. president confirmed this perception in
March 1953 before the AMA House of Delegates, when he
professed "certain philosophical bonds with doctors." Kaiser
lobbyist Chad Calhoun conveyed his "impression" to Henry
Kaiser that the secretary of the newly formed Department of
Health, Education, and Welfare (HEW), Oveta Culp Hobby,
was "working quite closely with the AMA" and would "no
doubt be greatly guided by it."[73]

Hobby stated her "personal philosophy" in a first press interview with the *New York Times*. Adequate medical care would
be achieved by "expanding and perfecting the system of voluntary, non-profit, privately operated health insurance programs." Like the president, she was "opposed to socialized
medicine." Hobby further assured her constituency that the
budget cut for the Public Health Service would be 19 percent,
or over $51 million.[74]

PHS and National Institutes of Health (NIH) spokespersons saw abandonment of an aggressive public health policy as
a critical blow to agency effectiveness. There were severe doctor and hospital bed shortages at the same time that illness cost
workers 400 to 500 million working days a year. Medical indi-
gence was still widespread. A third of the 46 million U.S.
dwellings had "basic health deficiencies." One in seven was
overcrowded, one in eleven "dilapidated," and almost one in
three without hot and cold running water. Almost 13,000
lacked even "decent toilet facilities."[75]

Ignoring these realities, Eisenhower Republicans accentuated domestic tranquility and the idyllic virtues of suburbia.
By 1955 70 percent of the nation's families purchased almost
eight million automobiles. The following year the government
launched the largest public works program in history, to build
thousands of miles of interstate highway that shattered the
geographic isolation of thousands of communities. Less than
17,000 television sets were in use in 1946; by 1953 two-thirds
of the nation's families owned one.[76]

Social welfare fell to the bottom of the domestic political

agenda. Even proposals by such Democrats as James Murray and Hubert Humphrey were moderate, asking extension of the 1935 Social Security Act for the disabled and elderly. Kaiser was interested in Republican measures focusing on tax incentives and construction loan guarantees for hospitals— facilities rather than increased medical care services. Republicans joined Democrats in bills to extend authorization of the $15 million annual Hill-Burton appropriations. Kaiser Washington lobbyist Chad Calhoun optimistically kept Kaiser abreast of these developments, focusing on the possibility for future government support of plans like Kaiser's in a $15 million "reinsurance" bill by Representative Charles A. Wolverton as H.R. 7700. The Wolverton bill would provide government guarantee of private sector loans for construction of medical facilities. Entitled the Hospital and Medical Facilities Mortgage Loan Insurance Act, it would protect private insurers against excessive loss and authorize self-liquidating FHA-style loans for construction. It differed from Hill-Burton in that it gave loan guarantees to private lenders rather than direct grants and allocations to the states. The new bill could give timely support for Kaiser's rapid $9 million to $12 million facilities expansion then under way. Moreover, Hill-Burton was based on state surveys and local commissions controlled by the AMA. The Wolverton proposal was based on the lay private sector.[77]

Hobby was a particular concern of Kaiser lobbyists. They courted her with cautious suspicion. In a private meeting in her office in January 1953, she delegated responsibility for passage of the hospital construction loan bill to Henry Kaiser. "That is a job you can do, Mr. Kaiser," she informed him, "better than anyone in government," but he would need "a groundswell of public acceptance" before he would "get an FHA type of hospital construction through Congress." She left it to Kaiser to create his own groundswell, aiming condescending remarks his way about relations with the AMA. "Everyone in this room wants better and lower cost medical care," she lectured him, "but, Mr. Kaiser, you are your own worst witness because you have been talking so much about AMA opposition. . . . They [AMA doctors] must be sold the idea it doesn't destroy their freedom or their initiative." They had to be shown that it "just isn't the socialized way." Kaiser had to do the selling without Hobby's aid. She refused even to give him names of potential supporters.[78]

Kaiser swallowed Hobby's scolding undaunted, even with a touch of obsequiousness. His staff eagerly sought signs of her approval by combing her public statements. Kaiser was adept at political gaming and curried her favor, personally trying to persuade her to visit California. Though they had to confer with Kaiser all the way from the East Coast, often to as far west as Kaiser's new headquarters in Hawaii, his lobbyists remained poised through the spring and summer of 1953 to throw the organization's support behind an appropriate government initiative. Kaiser himself continued to present his national plan at the opening of new facilities.[79]

Finally, at year's end, Republican Representative Wolverton asked Kaiser to help him prepare a bill to establish insured loans for hospitals and other medical facilities. Wolverton was demanding; he gave the Kaiser team only six weeks to complete a draft of the proposal while he was in Europe.[80] Then Wolverton became condescending. The bill drawn up by Kaiser's staff was not in proper form and appeared to be written by a doctor "who had about as much business drafting a legal document as a lawyer would have in writing a medical prescription." He directed Kaiser to rewrite it. Kaiser's deference to the politician paid off. He received favorable national press coverage for his support of the bill, and the president gave recognition to the Kaiser model in his state of the union address before he introduced his own health proposal. "I am flatly opposed to the socialization of medicine," said Eisenhower. "The great need for hospital and medical services can best be met by the initiative of private plans." He went on to endorse the reinsurance bill.[81]

But the HEW staff displayed little enthusiasm for Kaiser's involvement in national politics. The day after he testified before the congressional committee considering the bill, Kaiser met with a Hobby physician staff member. Frustrated with the tone of the hearing, Kaiser remarked, "This Administration is scared to death of the AMA." The doctor paused, then replied, "I hear the unions are very enthusiastic to your plans." "I see," Kaiser retorted, "that's what you're afraid of." Kaiser lobbyists viewed the appointment of a former AMA legal adviser as associate general counsel for HEW as final proof that the AMA was "entrenched" in the department.[82]

Labor leaders had a mixed, then negative reaction to the Wolverton bill. Kaiser appealed personally to Walter Reuther to support it, emphasizing that it stipulated that 75 percent of facilities built under the proposal would be prepaid medical plans operating on a group practice basis. This is where Kaiser diverged sharply from AMA conservatives. Group practice based on collective payment and distribution of fees totally corrupted the traditional doctor-patient relationship based on individual intimacy and trust. The HEW staff played down this aspect of the proposal, but it was essential to any support from labor. Reuther assured Kaiser that the UAW-CIO was not opposed to H.R. 7700, though he stressed union belief that only large government subsidies and a broad-based federal insurance program would create an equitable system. The AFL concurred with Reuther.[83]

Henry Kaiser made amazing odysseys back and forth from Hawaii to the East Coast, while his Washington lobbyists became an irritant to experienced politicos. It was increasingly clear that Kaiser's support was not helpful to the Wolverton coalition. Representative Wolverton told Kaiser adviser Robert Elliott in no uncertain terms to leave the politicking at HEW to him. Kaiser and his aides were asked to stick with cultivating their banking connections. But the bankers were even less enthusiastic about reinsurance than were the unions and HEW, and "Mrs. Hobby's Department" was increasingly stone faced in deliberations. Kaiser ignored signs that Wolverton was irked when the industrialist persisted in ill-advised correspondence with Nelson Rockefeller and other department members. Kaiser could not even influence the bankers. His old standby, the Bank of America, informed Trefethen that its board of directors did not favor loans to hospitals and had worked with Kaiser for two reasons only: Kaiser's other financial relations with the bank and the organization's proven prepaid plan.[84]

Kaiser made his last plea for the "new economics of medical care" before the National Press Club on 26 May 1954. Just as he had during the World War II, he stressed the shortcomings of the medical system in terms of lost manpower, now at $30 million a year. The cost to "the people" was even greater. In a single year small loan companies reported loans for medical expenses totaling over $480 million and charged interest averaging 33 percent per annum for an additional $84 million. Kaiser spoke eloquently on behalf of average Americans who wanted the best medical science offered for their families. "I can't understand for the life of me," he exclaimed in an exaggerated tone of shock, "why there should be any conflict or controversy over any plan that brings comprehensive high quality medical care to Americans at low cost, especially when that plan was carried out under the American free enterprise system. I *can* understand, and am completely in sympathy with those who would oppose any plan of *socialized medicine*, for I, too, have always been opposed to it." In reference to his plan to sponsor a Norman Vincent Peale program on national television, he concluded with a religious couplet that reflected the melding of Christianity, mass media, and patriotism popular among the politicians and public figures of the era:

> I sought to hear the voice of God,
> And climbed the topmost steeple,
> But God declared: "Go down again,
> I dwell among the people."[85]

Kaiser used the same populist language in confrontations with the AMA on the national level. Citing a string of AMA court defeats by prepaid group health plans following the GHA decision, Kaiser attributed AMA opposition to the desire for monopoly at the expense of the public interest.[86]

By midsummer, a month after the press club address, the stumbling blocks to Kaiser's national health plan were legion. They included his colleagues in private finance along with other "friends of the people" disillusioned with what Democratic leader Sam Rayburn called a "blundering, stupid way to start" a national health program. AMA spokespersons finally launched a "full counter attack" against Kaiser in committee hearings, calling H.R. 7700 the "Kaiser bill" and an aid "to bail out Henry Kaiser."[87] By early 1955 the American Hospital Association joined the AMA in accusations about a Kaiser "bailout." Ultimately the combination of administration foot-dragging and opposition by entrenched interests proved fatal for the health bill in the Eighty-third Congress. The small Republican majority succeeded in enacting less than a quarter of the president's domestic bills, none under the category of welfare and education.[88]

Creative with words, Chad Calhoun drew Kaiser a grim scenario of the "black cloud" of defeat on the Washington horizon. He attributed failure in the House not to political causes or to the larger socioeconomic issues that were the focus of the labor movement and the AMA, but to enmity toward the Kaiser organization. Calhoun believed that the "dark" rumor that the Wolverton bill was a "bailout" was perpetrated by congressional cohorts of Cyrus Eaton then in legal battle with Kaiser over a shady stock deal. Eaton sycophants included John L. Lewis, with whom Kaiser then had a rocky relationship.[89]

A final exchange in regard to the Wolverton bill revealed a core principle of Kaiser's national health plan that was unacceptable to the AMA but essential to Kaiser. Calhoun wrote that he had agreed to delete the stipulation that 60 percent of the loan guarantees under the bill be earmarked for group practice plans. This was already a large reduction from the 75 percent he had told Reuther. Kaiser was appalled. "Fundamentally you know that my whole purpose in life has been to get prepaid group practice nationally in order that more people could have better medicine at lower cost. How I could reverse this position or that you could feel that it was reversed or that you could let them feel that it was reversed is shocking." He warned that it might be necessary for him to journey to Washington to state his unaltered position before Rockefeller and "all of them."[90]

Henceforth Kaiser was irascible toward Washington politicos, refusing to entertain or even see those interested in his health plan when they visited Honolulu, where he lived. Health politics became a routine function of the corporate public relations, legal, and lobbying staff.[91]

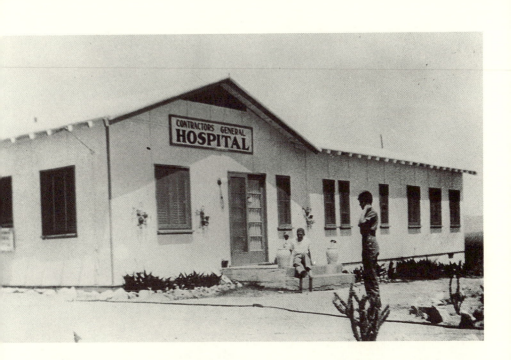

Fig. 1. Sidney R. Garfield, M.D., sits on the front step of his first hospital, Contractor's General, Desert Center, California, 1933 (other figure unidentified). Courtesy of Kaiser Permanente.

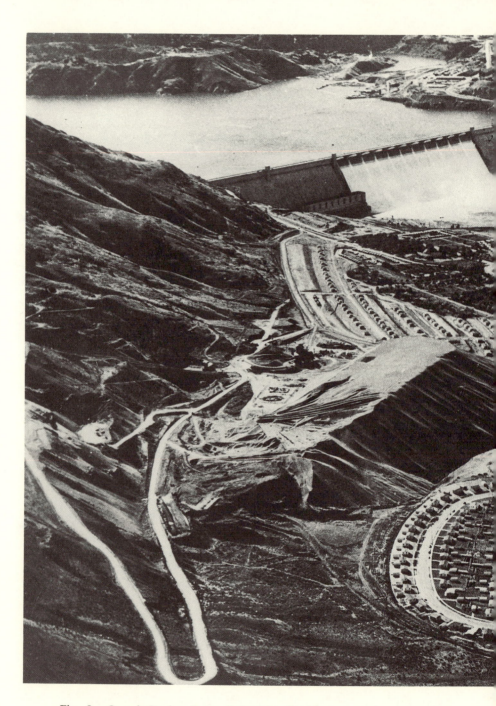

Fig. 2. Grand Coulee Dam, Columbia, Washington, and construction town, late 1930s. Courtesy of Kaiser Permanente.

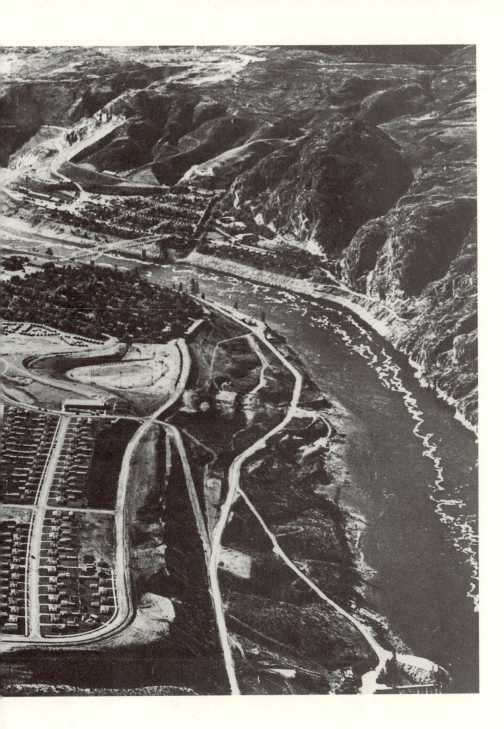

Fig. 3. Shipway, Kaiser shipyards, Richmond, California, early 1940s. Courtesy of Kaiser Permanente.

Fig. 4. In Richmond, probably 1942–1943, an outmoded bus is home for a family of six. Courtesy of The Bancroft Library (1983.019.46).

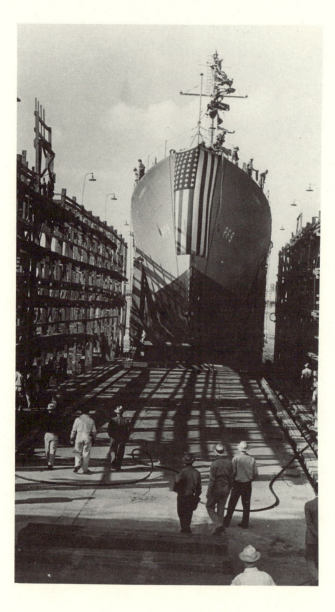

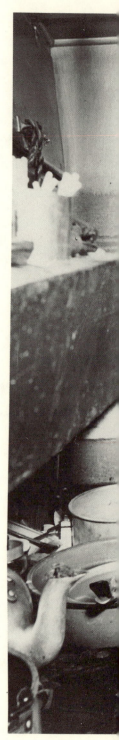

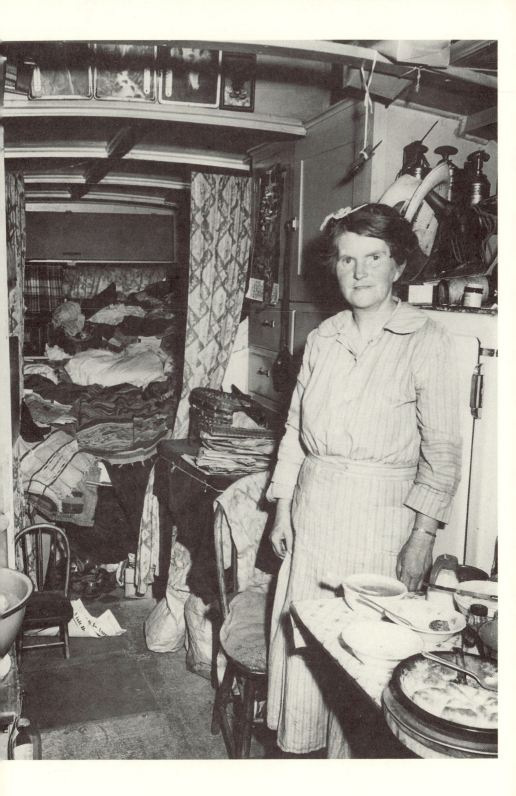

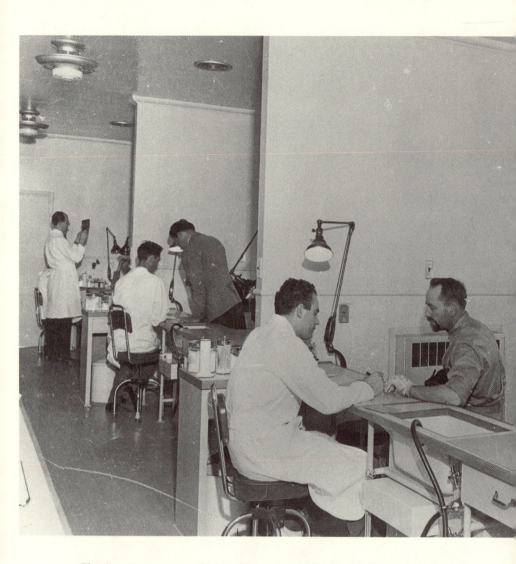

Fig. 5. Treatment cubicles, Richmond Field Hospital, c. 1942, feature semiprivacy. Note that the doctors are behind counters and that apparatus also is removed from contact with the patients. Courtesy of Kaiser Permanente and Eugene E. Trefethen, Jr.

Fig. 6. Eleanor Roosevelt visits a patient at Portland-Vancouver, with Edgar Kaiser in the background, 1943. Courtesy of The Bancroft Library (1983.069.163).

Fig. 7. A nurse pulls out a drawer so a mother can see her baby in a typical maternity room in the Kaiser Foundation Hospital, San Francisco, 12 February 1954. Other technology included "electric-motor type beds for automatic adjustment, build-in lavatory with hot, cold and ice water taps, five-channel radio, piped oxygen, individual toilets and clothes closets, telephone, over-bed dressing table, and electrically operated drapes." Courtesy of the ILWU Library, San Francisco.

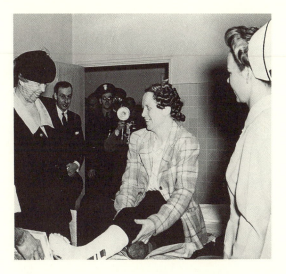

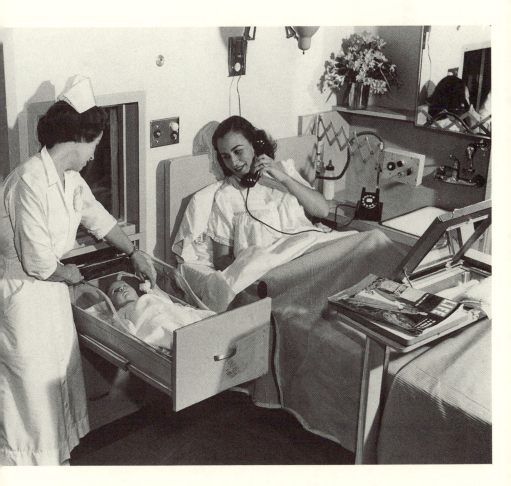

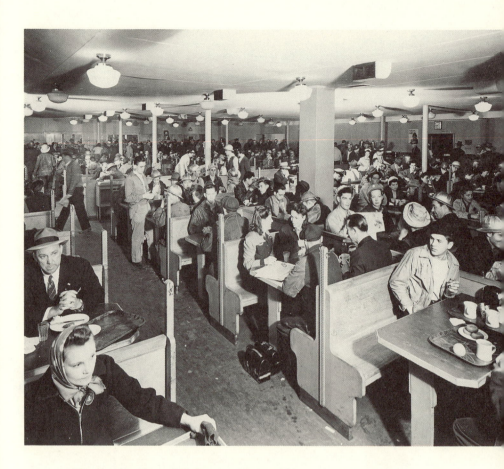

Fig. 8.   Employees' Cafeteria, Oregon Shipyard, 1941–1945. Courtesy of
The Bancroft Library (1983.020.167).

4 Henry Kaiser Takes Charge: Medical McCarthyism

In 1951 Henry Kaiser turned his energies and interest back to the Permanente medical program. He was at heart a builder rather than ideologue, and he preferred to focus on hospital construction rather than on the ethical controversies that swirled around him. In what top executives called a "unilateral" act, Kaiser directed the corporate trustees to give the Permanente hospitals and health plan the Kaiser name. His staff ordered new stationery and changed the names on existing facilities. The trustees directed that all future hospitals and those under construction have the Kaiser name "embedded in masonry or concrete."[1]

Kaiser also put his stamp on nearly every material aspect of the country's consumer culture of the 1950s: homes, kitchen gadgetry, automobiles, airplanes, and recreational equipment from jeeps, radio, and television to luxury cruisers and resort hotels.

He formed Kaiser Community Homes with developer Fritz Burns to join in the nation's postwar suburbanization. By 1950 suburban growth was tenfold more than that of established urban centers, as an estimated nine million people moved to suburban areas; by 1960 the suburbs had thirteen million more inhabitants than the core cities. Kaiser Community Homes built only one-fifth of 1 percent of the nation's new units between 1945 and 1950, with a total construction of under 10,000. Undaunted by the slow take-off of his housing market, for several years after the war Kaiser operated a "research and development" laboratory in Emeryville in the East Bay to test dishwashers, air conditioners, washer and drier combinations, kitchen ranges, vacuum cleaners, and lawnmowers. The domestic manufacturing and homebuilding ventures were centered in the three major West Coast regions where the health plan also burgeoned: Los Angeles, the San Francisco Bay Area, and Portland, Oregon. He headed dozens of companies, international and domestic, with assets of nearly $1 billion. Kaiser exited the war as the archetypal regionalist of his time and place in his contribution to a modern socioeconomic order on the variegated Pacific shoreline. His enterprises emerged organically from the regional topography, natural resources, and population.[2]

Decentralization into ambulatory and short-term care facilities and independent medical groups extended the health program deep into the scattered suburban and new urban centers of northern California. Not an intellectual, Kaiser probably was unversed in contemporary regional planning theory. Yet he early demonstrated urban theorist Lewis Mumford's idea of a "New Conservation," integrating natural resources and community values in regional development. Mumford echoed both Thomas Jefferson and Frederick Jackson Turner when he wrote that permanent agriculture, forestry, and human communities should supplant "land-skimming," "timber mining," "camps and squatter-settlements." "Stable buildings" should replace "the scantling and falsework of our 'go-ahead' communities."[3] The Kaiser dam and shipyard communities signified these stages. The health plan and artifacts of material culture Kaiser produced after the war represented community permanence.

He sought personal notoriety in these endeavors as the Kaiser nomenclature was finely tuned. The title "Foundation" was appended to "Kaiser" in the renaming of the hospitals.[4]

Foundation had the elevated connotation of private philanthropy in its association with the Carnegie, Rockefeller, and Ford foundations that Kaiser emulated, during a decade in which unprecedented public and private funds poured into the nation's premier teaching and research institutions. The National Institutes of Health was the primary distributor of government funding for medical research. Its budget leapt from $7 million in 1947 to $70 million by 1953, at the same time that federal legislation pumped funds through the states for hospital survey and construction. The emphasis on facilities, research, and education underlined the postwar belief in unlimited scientific progress to cure disease, overcome disability, and achieve a better quality of life.[5]

The Kaiser Foundation could make a significant regional impact. Western and southern schools were neglected by established benefactors. Only the Rockefeller General Education Board (GEB) made large grants to public institutions outside of the urban Northeast and elite specialists. Up to its demise in 1960 the GEB gave $94 million to twenty-four medical schools. Cornell, Chicago, Johns Hopkins, Vanderbilt, and Washington University in St. Louis received over half of board funds up to 1936. Institutions at the top of regional educational hierarchies such as Johns Hopkins, Stanford, and Vanderbilt were founded by businessmen in the late nineteenth century. The balance of power between philanthropic financial interests and physicians, however, remained a delicate issue in institutional control. Medical faculty were wary of large contributions from single lay sources.[6]

In his quest for legitimacy and recognition in elite medical circles, Kaiser had formidable rivals in the Bay Area, including Stanford Hospital and the University of California, San Francisco (UCSF), which in the 1950s asserted its own preeminence in the region. In 1947 UCSF broadly expanded research and teaching programs. With the generous NIH and other funding of the postwar decade, it opened new foundations and institutes in ophthalmology and cancer. In the early 1950s it expanded metabolic, radioactivity, and cardiovascular research. Construction of the medical sciences building and

Moffitt Hospital began in 1954 and 1955. The medical science classes at the Berkeley campus were moved back to San Francisco in 1952 after four decades of rivalry between the UC campuses in the West and East Bay, and enrollment at UCSF nearly doubled.[7]

In the late 1950s UCSF and Stanford effectively divided their regional medical education and research domain. Stanford Hospital (formerly the Cooper Medical College, and then Lane Hospital) retreated to its home campus in the South Bay from its nineteenth-century berth in the city, away from the spreading UC medical campus and student competition for scarce and badly managed hospital beds.[8] Kaiser Permanente kept and extended its presence in San Francisco. Despite the chronic oversupply of physicians and the Stanford and UC faculty, the fragmented hospital system in San Francisco did not offer adequate efficiently organized facilities and care for the middle economic levels of the urban population. After the war Kaiser Permanente moved to fill this gap in working-class and middle-income family care, launching its own multi-million dollar expansion program in the San Francisco Bay and Los Angeles metropolitan areas.

In the early 1950s West Coast academia was far from accepting the corporate monolith into its elite ranks. Even the railroad and transit magnate and senator Leland Stanford had failed in the late 1880s to gain an appointment to the UC Board of Regents. After the state legislature refused to confirm a promised position with the regents, Stanford opened his own university in 1891 in honor of his deceased son. Kaiser, too, stubbornly sought acceptance by the venerable academic institutions of the region. According to advisers who later commented on events, he wanted the "whole ball of wax," meaning to stamp an image on every aspect of medicine and health in his far western economic empire.[9] Ironically, the pragmatic Kaiser did not recognize that dichotomous needs were served by research-oriented academic institutions and by Kaiser Permanente clinical services for the union and wage-earning population in the port cities.

While Henry Kaiser's attention was on the West Coast academic elite, more practical problems erupted inside Kaiser hospital walls. The ILWU coastwide contract was signed on 9 February 1950, little more than a week after Joseph McCarthy's speech in Wheeling heralded an era of anticommunist hysteria nationally. The Kaiser trustees, dominated by Henry Kaiser, consistently opposed consumer or union participation in policy and management decisions. Nevertheless, pressure from these groups brought improvements. The ILWU contract, for example, eliminated the per-visit patient surcharges imposed to lower base subscription rates and compete with Blue Cross–Blue Shield. In southern California the union prompted establishment of outpatient services in San Pedro and Harbor City between 1949 and 1950, using community facilities until the Harbor City medical center was built in 1957. The Los Angeles program began at the request of the Retail Clerks with an outpatient clinic and construction of the 200-bed hospital there.[10]

Henry Kaiser had always refused to grant members a voice in program policy decisions. Yet even Kaiser recognized the inadequacy of the member complaint process. Administrators failed to keep careful records and follow up on problems. Only forty-eight complaints from a total membership of 170,000 were recorded by the end of 1952, going back for an unspecified period. "It is not impressive that no record has been kept of the phone complaints," Kaiser wrote to Garfield. How could administrators have any idea of member attitudes "without a record being established"? "Isn't it fully as important that you keep a record of the membership's attitude as it is that you keep a record of their illness on charts?"[11]

The ILWU persistently complained about the lack of member representation but also continued its strong support. Welfare officers did not proceed with a proposed union-run medical plan to replace Kaiser, though study of union health centers continued through 1957. The poor record of other unions made Kaiser more attractive. In a report for the Longshore Welfare Fund, ILWU secretary Goldie Krantz focused on the extensive litigation engaged in by the UMW with the medical societies of Pennsylvania, Ohio, and Colorado. Society opposition to prepaid group practice and control by organized labor severely retarded positive development of the Mine

Workers' medical program ten years after Lewis's health and retirement funds began. The main issue in litigation was the medical society declaration that any doctor who deviated from orthodox fee-for-service practice would be denied society membership. Resulting professional handicaps included denial of hospital privileges, of referrals, and even of board certification in certain specialties.[12]

John L. Lewis presided over the most militant of the industrial unions. By 1950 the UMW represented 416,000 workers, who mined 90 percent of the nation's coal. Lewis was health plan trustee as well as union president, with a power base constructed on health and welfare benefits. Lewis's actions on behalf of the medically destitute miners in the brutal coal regions of the Southeast paralleled expansion of Henry Kaiser's successful corporate-directed plan in the West. UMW Health Fund trustees sought to establish a complete medical service system for members in the Southeast but were stymied by entrenched medical interests in the region and by insufficient resources. Ultimately, Lewis and his associates were able only to expand the prepaid contract system that had evolved since the nineteenth century. They continued to deal inefficiently with doctors and substandard proprietary hospitals on an individual fee-for-service basis.[13]

Lewis took an active and controversial interest in Kaiser Permanente, encouraging Kaiser to undertake bold geographic expansion to the Southeast coal mining region. The initial motivation for their relationship was their mutual interest in neuromuscular disorders, suffered by Lewis's men and also by Kaiser's son. During the war, the Kaiser family discovered that Henry J. Kaiser, Jr., had multiple sclerosis. For this reason, as the Permanente Foundation Health Plan began to experience its period of phenomenal growth, the senior Kaiser decided to fund the clinical research of a young Washington, D.C., neurologist. Dr. Herman Kabat first gained a reputation with the U.S. Public Health Service. In 1946 he established the Kabat-Kaiser Institute, incorporated in 1948 as a nonprofit, charitable corporation funded by the Permanente Foundation. At that time there were fewer than fifty doctors in the United States qualified in physical rehabilitation, and the AMA had just created a Board of Physical Medicine in recognition of needs in the new field. The institute originally operated through facilities in the capital bought by the Permanente Foundation. It then expanded into space at the Vallejo, California, hospital leased in 1947 by Permanente for the navy's Mare Island workers, and then to its own building in Santa Monica, California.

By March 1949 the institute was treating over 300 cases of multiple sclerosis. At the same time the UMW prompted a more comprehensive rehabilitation program geared toward the needs of its members. When the UMW Welfare and Retirement funds were created in 1946, victims of mining accidents were sent for treatment of neurological injuries and paralysis at UMW fund expense to Vallejo from as far as the West Virginia coal fields. (Most Santa Monica patients were poliomyelitis victims.) In 1950 almost 200 patients in the capital, over 400 at Vallejo, and another 600 at Santa Monica were treated at institute units. The Kaiser organization early recognized the institute's public relations value, and Dr. Kabat encouraged "exploiting" its "dramatic human interest appeal" in the press. Coal miners placed out of the institute into positions in various Kaiser enterprises were highlighted in articles in popular periodicals.[14] Kaiser was sincere about treating the miners. When the union fund suffered a financial setback in late 1949, the Permanente Hospitals Foundation continued to transport and care for miners at Permanente expense. Kabat-Kaiser continued through 1952 to run on a deficit of almost $100,000.[15]

Kaiser's increased interest in medical affairs was intensely personal on another level as well, and not merely a bid for personal power. In 1951 Kaiser and Garfield became extremely close. Even as Henry Kaiser, Jr., was entering the last decade in his struggle with multiple sclerosis, Bess Kaiser, Henry Kaiser's wife of forty-three years, was on her deathbed, suffering from chronic nephritis. Because Kaiser did not want her to go into the hospital, Sidney Garfield and Cecil Cutting set up a miniature hospital in the Kaiser apartment in Oakland. Cutting, along with Garfield's head administrative nurse, Alyce Chester, moved into the apartment to care for

Bess Kaiser during her last six months. Cutting's main recollection of those months was of Henry Kaiser's daily hamburger barbecues and continual business talk, "mostly about things like using aluminum engines in cars." Bess Kaiser died in February 1951. Kaiser was a widower for little more than a month; on 10 April 1951 he married Alyce Chester. Associates have attributed his compulsion to dominate the medical program personally to that event and to "Ale" Kaiser's medical interests.[16] Kaiser's marriage to Garfield's nurse was symbolic of his attempted merger of the corporate and medical components of his industrial empire. His high national profile in medical reform continued to enhance his public image, even as it irritated the medical profession.

Kaiser tried many positive approaches to break down AMA enmity. As the rumblings of discontent by local doctors grew louder, he tried to force acceptance of Permanente at a higher level through a "Plan to Unite the AMA and Permanente" that he thought should be "rapidly realizable." In the philanthropic tradition of Carnegie and Rockefeller, his own Kaiser Foundation would offer grants and facilities to noted medical schools suffering financial problems. He chose the prestigious Stanford University Medical School as the object of his benefaction, offering to build a medical center adjacent to the medical school in San Francisco to train Stanford interns and residents and to serve Permanente patients. This would relieve the prestigious school from dependence on other sources for the astronomical sums necessary to provide its own research and patient facilities.[16] After 1929, financing shifted dramatically from private sources to government. Public spending on medical care and research increased from 13.6 percent to 27.2 percent between 1929 and 1950, rising steadily thereafter. Medical school expenses increased at an incredible rate, from $69.5 million in 1947 to $884 million in 1965, with approximately one-half from the federal government.[17]

Bacteriologist and popular medical writer Paul de Kruif assumed the role of mediator with AMA leaders to gain support for Kaiser's endeavor with Stanford. He persuaded AMA president-elect Dr. Elmer L. Henderson and AMA general manager Dr. George F. Lull to come to California to placate local medical leaders and effect a truce with Permanente. Whether Kaiser actually tried to avoid a meeting or was too busy to set a definite date, he would not commit to an appointment with the AMA leaders. The industrialist's rudeness angered de Kruif, who told Kaiser he would cancel all plans for the meeting.[18] Perhaps Kaiser remained angry at Garfield's persecutors and thought he could snub them with impunity. Perhaps the AMA leaders were seeking to buoy the status of local practitioners in the tough San Francisco medical market, while also boosting the influence of the county society. Whatever the motivations on each side, Kaiser's slight of the AMA officials permanently alienated de Kruif.

Kaiser and Trefethen preferred to deal directly with Stanford medical dean L. R. Chandler, though they must have known that Chandler was not an advocate of their prepaid group plan. Chandler was Cecil Cutting's former mentor who had advised Cutting not to join Garfield at Permanente.[19]

Kaiser and Trefethen deliberately avoided involving the AMA leaders in the approach to Chandler, preferring to deal on their own terms. At a dinner meeting that included Chandler, Kaiser, Trefethen, Garfield, and Cutting, Kaiser made the following proposal: Permanente would purchase property that was adjacent to Stanford's San Francisco medical school facilities for construction of a hospital and clinic. These facilities, costing $2.5 million, would be independent of Stanford, yet a complement to the medical school. Stanford, in turn, would provide medical service to Permanente patients in the clinic and hospital. This plan would save Stanford about $200,000 a year, but the benefits to Kaiser Permanente were even greater. It would relieve the pressure to recruit staff for rapidly expanding facilities. More importantly, it would bring long-sought professional legitimacy to the Permanente Medical Group. The top Kaiser echelon perhaps imagined that the prestige lent by the Stanford connection would crush the opposition of the California medical establishment.[20] (Kaiser's grandiose vision overwhelmed cautious physician leaders, who knew the industrialist's medical education goal was unobtainable in the 1950s and might further alienate their colleagues.)[21]

Chandler concluded the meeting on a negative note. Monetary advantages were a secondary concern. Before Stanford officials would even consider the Kaiser proposal, they needed answers to three questions: How would participation with the Kaiser Permanente form of practice affect the Stanford teaching philosophy? Would the financial savings promised be realized? Finally, what public relations problems might result from an association with Permanente? Rather than address the ideological and professional issues raised by Chandler, Trefethen closed the session by pressuring him for a business decision. Permanente already had acquired, he said, other San Francisco property to build a hospital. Because detailed planning of the new facility had been delayed pending the outcome of the Stanford partnership agreement, he requested a prompt decision on the partnership.[22]

Six months later the plan remained stalled. Kaiser's interest waxed and waned as other issues, events, and problems surfaced, but Trefethen kept the grand strategy smoldering. He wisely delegated authority for continuing negotiations to the Permanente doctors themselves. He gave the rather awesome responsibility to assuage the sensitivities of Stanford and local medical society officials to Dr. Richard Bullis from Los Angeles, whose father was on the California Board of Medical Examiners during the time of Garfield's ethics case. Trefethen finally recognized that the medical school faculty was not interested in developing a relationship with Kaiser. He encouraged Bullis to work through nonmedical university sources, again trying to circumvent the profession.[23]

By the end of 1952 Trefethen's hopes for the Stanford affiliation had dwindled considerably. He pursued other avenues into the medical education field. Others in the organization explored alternatives such as grants to "selected universities" for education and research focused on prepaid group medical care.[24] Stanford officials let the Kaiser plan die by inaction. Kaiser's legal counsel Scott Fleming later declared that Henry Kaiser was a "megalomaniac" in his desire to control the regional medical establishment. His answer to AMA and local society opposition was "to create his own universe." Others knew it was "mythology"; though the views of the physicians and faculty "ranged from total hostility to subtle hostility to wild-eyed radicals who thought we might do it." Not even Kaiser could break into academic medicine. Yet he was persistent. For several years after Kaiser Permamente's Hawaii region was established in 1958, Kaiser also explored the possibility of a Hawaiian medical school in partnership with the state government. One executive noted that the rest of the leadership was "foot-dragging, but did not want a confrontation with Mr. Kaiser about it."[25]

Two years after the initial flurry of activity, Kaiser continued to express personal interest in an association with Stanford or with the University of California. The Kaiser Foundation established a $100,000 grant program in northern California as well as with the University of Southern California and the University of California School of Nursing. The Kaiser Foundation hospitals also conducted intern and resident programs, especially successful with UCSF, whose own school of nursing was established in 1947.[26] But Kaiser had reached the limits of his personal power. Sharing with other private institutions the difficulty of establishing viable medical training schools, even Kaiser eventually closed the doors of the nursing school. Competition, recruitment difficulties, and more stringent licensing requirements made it impossible to compete with four-year academic programs.[27]

The focus on improving relations with the medical establishment drifted further into the background of corporate thinking. Garfield worked with corporate officials on other ways to enhance the prestige of the Permanente physicians. Energies were funneled so intensely into the practical matters of facility construction, physician recruitment, and day-to-day administration that physician executives could not devote sufficient time to the more exotic research and education initiatives required to gain full-fledged legitimacy in the medical establishment. Permanente clinicians were leaders in incorporating new antibiotics and treatment methods for pneumonia, venereal disease, and other diseases associated with occupational medicine. Conversely, the chronic "diseases of the affluent" were the major research fields at UCSF and other prestige institutions in the 1950s, and the affluent made up the major paying population for U.S. hospitals.[28]

The formal academic partnership sought by Kaiser was not

implemented. But Morris Collen developed successful cooperative programs with UCSF based on his own experiences at the University of Minnesota, where the Mayo Foundation had developed an affiliated graduate school of medicine. Thus the clinic that was the site of the first formal group practice in the United States achieved academic recognition for its innovative mode of organization. Collen persisted in giving an academic flavor to the organization through the *Permanente Foundation Medical Bulletin*. Permanente doctors received recognition for their expertise in treating pneumonia and acute diseases, to which UCSF students had little exposure at the university. The group also set up an intern rotation system at Oakland under the UCSF chair of the Department of Medicine, Dr. William Kerr. In 1958 a Kaiser Foundation Research Institute was established at Richmond, though it was short-lived. Kaiser-Permanente leaders trimmed their expectations of what the organization could contribute to clinical and health services research once they realized that significant research in the basic sciences required a medical school environment.[29]

Garfield was unable to keep a hand in every level of program administration, much less to implement research projects. Several short-lived cancer studies with European physicians ended with foreign doctors absorbed in petty jealousies and angry about inadequate support.[30] It seems that Garfield and Kaiser were not adept at judging the quality and potential of such projects. Kaiser sharply criticized the reports he received from the researchers, charging that goals were too abstract, budgets imprecise.[31]

Yet one significant clinical experiment with the ILWU was recognized by noted public health academicians. Its success underlined the Kaiser Permanente contribution to medical care organization rather than to biomedical laboratory research. In 1951 a multiphasic screening program emerged naturally from the vast experience in industrial medicine and the application of public health and preventive medicine. Aggressive union leadership stimulated the high degree of participation that made it effective. Harry Bridges and welfare fund secretary-treasurer Goldie Krantz were determined to change the poor health habits of longshoremen and to overcome their view of medical screening as a threat to their job security. Traditional anxieties about company doctors and corporate intrusion into private lives continued to operate against preventive medicine. Bridges forced his men to get their comprehensive physicals with the threat of "pulling the plug" on their employment.[32] He also assured the men that their jobs were secure regardless of the results of the exams, and that records were confidential. To further allay their fear the union and public agencies operated the project. Kaiser kept a low profile, with initial direction provided by Dr. E. Richard Weinerman, Garfield's new assistant from Yale University and an outspoken friend of unionism. Morris Collen, Cecil Cutting, Ernest Saward, and other Permanente leaders interested in clinical methods development later assumed responsibility.

The longshoremen profile made them a receptive group for the multiphasic experiment. They were cohesive and intensely loyal to the union despite their broad cultural and geographic diversity. The median age of the all-male group was forty-nine because attrition was extremely low after the contracts gained in the 1930s waterfront strike. At the same time medical problems were more pronounced than in younger groups with less arduous occupations.

The model preventive medicine program had excellent results because of the commitment to clinical experiment by Kaiser Permanente and the energetic community and union involvement. A spectrum of procedures was continually refined to screen large numbers in a short time. In one day several thousand men were tested for syphilis, tuberculosis, diabetes, cardiovascular disease, vision, hearing, and overweight. The twofold goals were to identify conditions not previously known, and to encourage treatment of those known but not treated. These goals were met, and the follow-up rate was high. More than 65 percent of the ILWU men in the Bay Area participated. Of these 4,000, two-thirds had positive screening tests, with 773 new diagnoses confirmed. Of the total diagnosed, 72 percent sought and received medical care for their conditions within four months.[33]

Despite Kaiser Permanente's successes with the unions and

achievements in clinical methods, preventive medicine, and outpatient care exemplified by the multiphasic screening program, medical educators in northern California refused to enter an alliance with Kaiser. The local medical societies continued to irritate the industrialist and stepped up harassment of the Permanente doctors.[34] Professional problems simply would not give way to Kaiser bullying. Caught in a conundrum of domestic politics and collegial hostilities, doctors inside and outside the organization were increasingly alienated by Kaiser's intrusive actions and high profile. AMA county society leaders ridiculed the Permanente doctors, whom they said worked for Henry Kaiser, and attacked Kaiser for unethical corporate interference in medical practice. The local medical societies rejected applications by Permanente doctors for membership and implied that they championed socialized medicine. Health plan doctors, in turn, resented Kaiser's personal meddling in medical affairs, which deprived them not only of professional autonomy within the health program but also of the respect of their peers. Mounting internal stresses between Kaiser and the doctors nearly shattered the program's integrity during its peak of expansion at midcentury. The doctors were trapped between the negative poles of Kaiser's autocracy and of rejection by their traditionalist colleagues.

When Kaiser put his name on the health plan and hospitals, Garfield elected Raymond Kay to confront the corporate magnate with the news that the doctors refused to be known as "Kaiser doctors." Although Garfield insisted that the name be confined to the health plan and hospitals, that the medical groups retain the title Permanente, he admitted he was "not getting anywhere" with "the Boss." At a meeting in Kaiser's large conference room only Kaiser, Trefethen, Garfield, and Kay huddled around its "giant table." Kay explained the doctors' objection to Kaiser. "Our Southern California partnership felt that we could not justifiably oppose the use of the names Kaiser Health Plan and Kaiser Hospitals, but we were very opposed to being labelled as the Kaiser Medical Group," he wrote later. "There had already been the insinuation by organized medicine that we worked for Mr. Kaiser, and we did not in any way want to give credence to that concept."[35] Kay told Kaiser that to be called the "Kaiser Medical Group . . . would just hurt us even more. . . . It would give truth to that lie that we were just [Kaiser doctors]." Trefethen agreed with the doctors' point about loss of collegial status. Kaiser retorted that "of course" he also agreed. Always one to get in the last word, he added, "I wouldn't let 'em use my name."[36] At least the issue was settled.

Northern California medical director Cecil Cutting was less charitable than Kay. According to Cutting, "Mr. Kaiser, a master industrialist, was also a compulsive, possessive manager. . . . He expressed his basic philosophy as anything he is a part of, he runs." Cutting did not agree with Kay that Kaiser and Trefethen capitulated to the medical group's demand so easily. "I don't think the Kaiser people were anxious to separate the medical group. . . . I think they wanted to assimilate the medical group."[37]

Months after signing its coastwide contract with Kaiser in 1950, the CIO ousted the ILWU for suspected Communist allegiance. The juxtaposition of these events created a paradox: Henry Kaiser, a towering and aggressive U.S. capitalist, built a prepaid group practice medical program supported by labor's left wing during one of the most reactionary periods in twentieth-century domestic politics. Permanente physicians also came under scrutiny for alleged Communist associations. Although the physicians shared Kaiser's pragmatic goal of broadening access to care, they also shared a social philosophy much closer to that of labor radicals than of corporate trustees. They engaged in corporate group practice because they sought income and family security—the bread-and-butter issues of the labor movement. Doctors in Portland and Vancouver and in Vallejo in northern California were farthest left of the centrist position in the Kaiser board room. Disabled UMW members came to the Permanente hospital and rehabilitation institute at Vallejo from as far as the West Virginia coal fields for long-term treatment. Several Vallejo physicians went well beyond a liberal sympathy with the civil rights movement in their identification with Marxism and the Communist party. On the other hand, Permanente leaders regarded Henry

Kaiser as staunchly anticommunist. He had always insisted that the health plan was a protection against socialized medicine.

Kaiser's anticommunist politics did not appease local AMA doctors. They portrayed Permanente physicians as employees who acquiesced in the corporate practice of medicine by a layperson. Moreover, just as Kaiser's German heritage and corporate triumph conjured for some an image of the country's World War II fascist enemies, the union associations and socialist leanings of some Permanente physicians evoked fear of Sovietism.[38]

Kaiser's treatment of Permanente doctors as if they were members of his industrial labor force resembled the practices of tough labor leaders such as Bridges and Lewis. A Kaiser corporate attorney later observed that "Henry Kaiser hoped to control the doctors just as he controlled his manufacturing and other operations."[39] He wanted them to toe the corporate line, did not recognize their professional anxieties, and often expressed "shock" or "disbelief" that their generous compensation did not satisfy them. In the early 1950s Kaiser salaries were $25,000 to $30,000 for top doctors and averaged $18,500 for Permanente partners. These incomes compared favorably with those of doctors in private practice, who averaged under $13,500.[40]

A $12 million Kaiser expansion program paralleled membership growth, and Henry Kaiser loomed ever larger in program direction. The independent AMA physicians now sought to halt the amoebalike spread of the health plan. They rejected the applications of group plan doctors for membership in local medical societies, which in turn blocked their access to referral networks, privileges in independent hospitals, and certification by specialty boards. The Kaiser Foundation struck back by building, owning, and controlling all of its medical facilities. Moreover, the regional work force of union, government, and other employees served as a ready-made membership base for the foundation. For Permanente physicians the only real problem was thus the medical society barrier to obtaining specialty certification.

Kaiser first attacked the problem by assigning Dr. Richard Bullis, Jr., whose father had been on the Board of Medical

Examiners at the time of Garfield's indictment in the 1940s, to monitor how the applications of Permanente doctors for membership in medical societies were treated. Bullis, who was from southern California where he later returned to private practice, in September 1952 reported that the doctors were denied membership either outright by the admissions committees or by the committees' refusal to act upon applications. This was the tactic used by the Alameda–Contra Costa County Medical Society at Oakland, the San Francisco County Medical Society, the Solano County Medical Society at Vallejo, and the San Bernardino County Medical Society at Fontana. At Vallejo only one Permanente doctor was admitted to the Solano County society after 1945, and that occurred when he was in private practice and not yet with Permanente. A Permanente physician who was president of the California Society of Allergy and chair of the Allergy Section of the California State Medical Association was especially difficult for Solano to turn down when he applied for transfer from Los Angeles. An entire Solano business session was devoted to a discussion of his application, which then was "tabled" along with those of several others. Applicants were sometimes rejected with no other explanation than that they had obtained "insufficient votes." Those Permanente doctors who successfully gained admission through transfer from other societies or before the rejection policy was being fully implemented by the winter of 1952 were denied notice of society meetings and excluded from all fraternal activities.[41]

Because specialty boards in orthopedics, ophthalmology, and obstetrics/gynecology required medical society membership as a prerequisite for certification, denial of membership proved a serious hardship to Permanente doctors and patients. The program's large block of industrial workers and the focus on family medicine in the 1950s placed these specialties in great demand. Of the 125 full-time Permanente doctors in Oakland and San Francisco, 60 eligible for board admission in 1952 were not yet accepted. Individual examples of the exclusion policy abound. A Permanente doctor eligible for the military draft was rejected by the San Francisco County Medical Society and then denied certification by the

American Board of Internal Medicine. This rejection deprived him of prestige, status, opportunity for advancement, and the extra income these would bring. Two obstetrician/gynecologists were rejected by the Alameda County Medical Society and subsequently not allowed to take the board examinations because "they were not well enough known in their respective communities." The American College of Surgeons rejected one Permanente applicant not because of academic or professional shortcomings, but because he did not belong to the San Francisco Medical Society (SFMS), which had rejected him for his "association with Permanente," and the uncertain "relationship of the applicant to his confreres."[42]

The extent of the discrimination shook Bullis. In his report to Kaiser he accused the AMA societies and specialty boards of libel, monopoly, and restraint of trade. The most "obvious libelous falsehood," he stated, was contained in a report by medical journalist Paul de Kruif. In July 1951 SFMS president Dr. John Cline told de Kruif that one of the three doctors recently rejected by the San Francisco Medical Society was "a Communist or a strong leftist." Falling into step with the repressive anticommunist sentiment of the period, Kaiser executives had their own Permanente doctors investigated by the Western Research Association, described by advisers as a "reliable organization and best way to check on questions of loyalty." The research firm uncovered no evidence of communism or "leftist leanings" by any of the three doctors implicated. Bullis concluded that "Dr. Cline's forces" used false charges to provoke legal combat in order to "besmear" the health plan in court.[43]

Bullis's conclusion was accurate. Cline's main enemy was Henry Kaiser. The SFMS president told journalist Paul de Kruif that the industrialist would "waste his money" if he initiated a court fight against the society for not accepting Permanente doctors. Cline reminded de Kruif, who passed the statement along to Kaiser, that "the Society has the right to reject doctors if it doesn't like the way the doctors comb their hair or tie their shoes."[44]

Henry Kaiser's personal involvement in controversies with the local societies embarrassed health plan doctors and provoked the societies to retaliate. Kaiser's high profile in national politics added another level of stress for the doctors. While Senator Joseph McCarthy hurled false charges in the halls of Congress against alleged subversives in government, academia, and the performing arts, the Federal Bureau of Investigation (FBI) took notice of the left-wing politics of some Permanente doctors. The chief of medicine at Oakland in 1952 and 1953, Dr. Morris F. Collen, surmised that federal investigators wanted Kaiser to rout out physicians who were Communist sympathizers because of sensitive military installations such as Travis Air Force Base, Mare Island Naval Shipyard, Alameda Naval Air Station, and San Francisco Naval Shipyard at Hunter's Point. More than 6,000 civilian employees at these installations were Kaiser members in 1951 (table 2.2).[45]

Antisubversives saw a connection between leftist politics within Permanente and Communist infiltration of CIO unions. The Kabat-Kaiser Institute and hospital at Vallejo treated UMW members with neuromuscular disorders from the mines of West Virginia, Tennessee, and Kentucky. It was a locus of left-wing physicians. Collen later recalled that Vallejo medical director Dr. Leslie Collins was an "open Communist" who tried to get other doctors to join the party. Collins invited Collen, Garfield, and several other associates to an "evening affair" that turned out to be a Communist rally. Collen recalled that it "scared the hell" out of him. He subsequently learned the FBI recorded the licenses of cars parked at "these affairs" and that "somebody at the Kaiser office would keep track of us, and any physician we hired would be screened by the FBI to see if he had Communist affiliations."[46]

Henry Kaiser instituted his own corporate loyalty oath, which resembled the federal Employees' Loyalty Program administered by the FBI.[47] Parodying the federal program, Kaiser ordered that "loyalty to our government of all Permanente employees must be established beyond question." He required that Permanente physicians and staff take a "loyalty oath" to the United States.

No person will knowingly be accepted or continued as an employee whose loyalty to the United States government is not established to the satisfaction of Permanente. . . . The fact that a doubt exists regarding the loyalty of an individual, whether such doubt exists because of the individual's poor judgment or intention, will make employment or the continuance thereof with this organization impossible.[48]

In October 1951 the American Civil Liberties Union (ACLU) informed Kaiser that its northern California branch was "deeply disturbed by the impression, now spreading through the community, and confirmed by conference with your officials, that you have assumed a judicial and punitive authority over your employees." The ACLU director called Kaiser "disloyal" for flagrant violation of the political freedom granted by the U.S. Constitution. "If your procedures were generally adopted by employing enterprises throughout the country, they would bring about the setting up of hundreds or thousands of private loyalty courts . . . [that would] condemn American citizens to public disrepute . . . [and] deprive them of their means of livelihood."[49] Unmoved, Kaiser went on to seek control over even the doctors' personal activity during off-duty hours.

Dr. Herman Kabat, director of the Kabat-Kaiser Institute, left Vallejo for private practice abruptly in 1954. Although available sources provide no record of the reason for his departure, a chronicler of the Permanente Medical Group in northern California states that the "concern in the Kaiser organization about employing Communists or sympathizers . . . cost" Kabat his job. The title of the institute was changed, eliminating his name.[50] Dr. Ephraim Kahn was relieved of his position as Vallejo chief of medicine after he refused to sign the Kaiser oath.

Among the left-wing physicians visible in the northern California group was E. Richard Weinerman, a union health ideologue whose allegiance lay with the leftist Bay Area union welfare movement rather than with the firmly centrist Kaiser corporate boardroom. Weinerman left his post as a visiting professor of medical economics at the University of California School of Public Health when he refused to sign a state-mandated "loyalty oath" for faculty. He was asked to resign his post at Kaiser Permanente for the same reason and left the organization within a year amid charges that he was "disloyal" to the U.S. government, perhaps because of his union connections. Weinerman also refused to sign the Kaiser oath.[51]

Physicians interviewed later in regard to the political turmoil of the early 1950s suggested that a few Permanente doctors were under suspicion merely because they were civil rights activists. Kahn and others were active in the National Association for the Advancement of Colored People and Civil Rights Congress. Also, the ILWU considered both Kahn and Weinerman to be Kaiser insiders who gave the union information on racial and political discrimination inside Kaiser facilities.[52]

When Kahn was relieved of his duties for off-duty political activities and refusal to sign the Kaiser oath, a distressed former patient wrote Kaiser on his behalf, emphasizing the individual attention he gave his patients and his excellent medical work. The patient was shocked, as were others, she said, that a man with a family was given short notice to leave because of his beliefs "in high ideals of freedom and equality for all men." The writer called Kaiser's action "a new low in ethics." "I earnestly hope," she concluded, "that Permanente Hospitals are not becoming a political machine which will demand loyalty oaths of doctors just to keep in fashion with the hysteria that now engulfs us."[53]

ILWU officers were distressed by the drop in the quality of care at Kaiser, and about racial and political discrimination practiced at Kaiser facilities. Local 6 called a special meeting to decide what should be done "to bring pressure against Permanente Hospital, which would result in the hospital discontinuing discrimination and its refusal to accept Negro applicants for internships and other staff functions." It was attended by Dr. Kahn and representatives from black action groups as well as by union activists. The conferees were militant in their approach to problems uncovered through an informant in a "position of trust and authority in Permanente" who gave information to the Civil Rights Congress in regard to financial status and employment applications. This source may have been Weinerman, as he was referred to as a source of such information in an ILWU meeting on the subject.[54] Kahn reported from this source that the hospital had made a profit every month.

Kahn reported that a black intern, Dr. Wendell Lipscomb,

was "told he would have to go" a month after he began work
in Vallejo because in 1947 he had gone as a youth delegate
from the Unitarian church on a peace mission to Prague. Collen and Garfield talked Kaiser out of firing Lipscomb because
it would bring negative publicity. Another speaker at the
union meeting was a white Permanente orderly who reported
that when a woman objected to her husband being placed in a
room with a black patient who was an ILWU member, the
black ILWU member was "removed." The orderly called the
ILWU Welfare Committee to report the incident and was
fired (though later rehired) by Head Superintendent Nurse
Daniels. Reportedly Daniels was "hysterical" over the fact that
the orderly had "incited the patient" and was "calling in outside organizations, disrupting the work of the hospital, going
contrary to hospital policy, and being a troublemaker."[55] The
ILWU representative commented that if the union was going
"to put up the money and the memberships to support it, they
were going to have a say in how the hospital was run."

Collen described Henry Kaiser as vehemently anticommunist but not racist in these incidents. Another doctor noted
that Sidney Garfield believed Permanente already had an up-
hill battle for acceptance by traditional physicians. He told the
doctors that "it was enough to try to fight our own battles,
without trying to take on somebody else's fights at the same
time."[56]

The ILWU at this time also supported the United Public
Workers of America Local 722, then threatening to strike
against Permanente Hospital for its antiunion activities, specifically for the "mass firing of Attendants and Aides."[57] Union
members and others present at the meeting set the following
goals:

1.   To get a commitment from DR. GARFIELD that there would be
no discrimination in screening applicants for staff physicians in the
intern and resident class.
2.   That they solicit the aid of the ILWU and other large unions
holding membership in Permanente for the purpose of setting up a
long range program of control to get a hiring hall plan for all Permanente employees.
3.   That they be permitted to operate freely within the hospital re-

garding grievances of outside patients, or patients other than union members who might feel that their treatment was not up to what they thought was standard.[58]

All of these goals were unacceptable to Kaiser, who objected to consumer or union representation in medical program direction. Nevertheless, the ILWU set up an elaborate grievance procedure and continued pressure on Kaiser Permanente to create a joint committee with the union to discuss policy and procedures. Kaiser officials delayed sending a representative to the committee; Garfield himself tried to defuse the issue. The union continued its monitoring activities, following up on member complaints.[59]

Sidney Garfield was unable to maintain firm direction of the medical care program he had created. Although Kaiser intended Garfield to remain as the top lieutenant under his new personal management regime, Kaiser's meddling, physician anger and dissention, and the enormous geographic expansion in the early 1950s fatally undermined the doctor's administrative control. He could not protect the doctors in the Permanente Medical Group from the many controversies that developed during the McCarthy era on the national front or from Kaiser's intrusions into local affairs. Those who worked closely with Garfield from the beginning to the end of his tenure noted his personal administrative shortcomings that exacerbated interorganizational tensions. His attempt, along with Kaiser, to run the organization in their traditional manner, in spite of its size and the requirements of modern science, was ludicrous to close observers. Garfield certainly was not abreast of modern management techniques. One top executive recalled that even when membership grew beyond 250,000 he "was likely to jot down the agenda for meetings on the back of an envelope," and ran the program like a "Ma and Pa grocery store."[60]

By the middle of 1951 the large Permanente membership in northern California was served by the 300-bed central Oakland hospital and health center staffed by sixty-five full-time Permanente Medical Group doctors, by smaller hospital centers in San Francisco, by Richmond and Vallejo with an average of 40 to 100 beds and fifteen full-time doctors, and by outlying diagnostic clinics in Napa (opened by Dr. Joseph Moore formerly at Vallejo) and South San Francisco. In the Oregon region were a 250-bed hospital (with only 60 beds in use by Kaiser Permanente patients) and the clinic in Portland operated by twelve physicians. In southern California the 85-bed Fontana Hospital was staffed by twelve doctors, a clinic in San Pedro by five, and a new medical center in Los Angeles by fourteen. Large hospitals were planned for Los Angeles and San Francisco. Central purchasing, uniform record systems, and coordinated administration and financing were vital to the smooth operation of this enormous medical care network.[61]

By most accounts Garfield was unsuited for the management task. For one thing expansion added a new dimension to financing the program. Until the early 1950s funds largely were self-generating. Now huge sums were borrowed, and Garfield did not impress bankers as a good financial manager. Oregon medical director Ernest Saward observed that he ran "a very parsimonious organization" with a great deal of the bookkeeping "in his head." Henry Kaiser, on the other hand, had a very clear sense of how he wanted the program run—just like his steel, cement, and aluminum plants. This was done by measuring and projecting use of hospital beds and physician services for given member populations, and by carefully balancing the staff-to-patient ratio. By the early 1950s Kaiser realized that Garfield "wasn't a good businessman and he wasn't an organizer."[62] Nor was he always personable with staff physicians. "Sidney was a quiet individual," recalled his close colleague Cecil Cutting. "They'd think he was stuck up. But he was thinking about something else more important . . . he didn't mean to be unfriendly, but he was shy."[63]

Garfield and the trustees brought in a public health and union health movement advocate as an adviser and troubleshooter to iron out program deficiencies. Though virtually no mention is made in company records of his one-year tenure as Garfield's "assistant," Dr. E. Richard Weinerman made interesting observations in his own papers that illuminate the reasons for the turmoil and the daily conflicts that occurred during the McCarthy era among Permanente physicians and at Kaiser Foundation facilities. In a confidential report to Garfield, he fulfilled his assignment to identify problems within the medical program that provoked complaints by doctors and members. He targeted as unsatisfactory the excessive control of medical policy by Garfield and Kaiser Foundation trustees (primarily the Kaisers and Gene Trefethen), general administration, member relations, and quality of medical care—in other words, every aspect of the program. He cited wildly fluctuating levels of quality in facilities and among departments, overloaded physicians, and the "mass" or assembly-line aspects of prepaid group practice designed to serve large numbers at the lowest possible cost as reasons for the substandard doctor-patient relations and quality of care.[64]

Control of medical policy by Kaiser executives was autocratic and undemocratic, charged Weinerman. "The overlapping Boards of Trustees of Health Plan, Hospitals and Foundation do dominate overall program policy, with Dr. Garfield as the single strong maker and administrator of policy." Weinerman believed strongly that the board "in a nonprofit community health agency should be broadly representative of the whole community, and not composed only of officials of one industry." Yet membership in Kaiser Permanente was not represented in Health Plan policy and "constructive handling of grievances" was "rare."[65]

In a final indictment Weinerman told Garfield that internal administration of the program was "archaic and unwieldy at the higher levels. Clear lines of authority and responsibility, proper definition of function, and consistent administrative planning are not in evidence." Nor was there "democratic staff organization, planning conferences," or development of an "informal liaison with employees." He concluded that the result of these severe shortcomings in a program that purported to serve "the people" and to provide a national private enterprise model was the obvious member and staff dissatisfaction that had surfaced, and "waste, delay, frustration and impaired productivity." Attached to a draft of Dr. Weinerman's report in his own file was a typescript of the loyalty oath referred to by the ACLU, designed by the executive board for health program staff, and for which Dr. Kahn had just been dismissed. Weinerman made handwritten question marks all over the oath demanding to know "for whom," "how" and what "Kaiser criteria" would be used in the corporate attempt to "subvert" political freedom within the walls of Kaiser facilities.[66]

Weinerman departed within a year of his arrival, simultaneously with the ACLU charges against Kaiser and amidst rumors of Weinerman's own "disloyalty." His report to the trustees about program fallacies was only part of the problem he presented for program directors. Garfield in northern California, Raymond Kay in the south, and other executives scurried around after Weinerman's disclosures in an attempt to close the Pandora's box he had unlatched. In southern California Kay hastily patched up trouble the outspoken Weinerman stirred up with the unions, the Retail Clerks in particular.

In talks with Retail Clerks' union president Joe DeSilva and other union leaders, Weinerman apparently sought their help in remedying problems at Kaiser Permanente and gave De-Silva clear reasons for his pending resignation. First on the list was the fact that Kaiser himself was personally responsible for the discharge of the "colored orderly" (actually white, according to union records) who had reported discrimination to the union—the issue over which the ILWU and ACLU continued to agitate. According to Weinerman, Kaiser's interference was the root of all difficulties. "Profit consciousness" and facility expansion were the industrialist's primary goals, he thought, to the detriment of quality medical care. Because the trustees were pouring more money into facilities and a decreasing proportion into service, the medical quality in northern California was on the "downgrade," and less competent physicians were employed. Even Garfield had "fallen" excessively under the magnate's "influence," Weinerman told DeSilva, regarding "concessions" to the AMA and CMA. Because of these circumstances "the unions up north were considering setting up their own Health Plan," he informed the union leader. Finally, Weinerman said, he was "quite worried" that Permanente might label him a "Red" and thus ruin his own career. After hearing of these allegations, Kay arranged a meeting with DeSilva, Weinerman, and Garfield to air grievances before the "accusations" spread to other unions.[67]

The day after Kay informed Garfield of the discontent Weinerman was spreading to the unions, Weinerman gave a farewell address to the Permanente doctors in northern California to which a distraught Garfield offered an emotional rebuttal. After a period of debate over which doctors would be permitted to attend Weinerman's presentation—only partners in the medical group, or nonpartner staff doctors as well—Weinerman launched into an impassioned defense of his position. His objections to program operation were decidedly not those of the traditionalists in organized medicine. He had come, he assured his listeners, as a "prior convert" to the precepts of full-time group practice, comprehensive family care, and prepayment, which he felt were uniquely implemented at Kaiser Permanente on an unprecedented scale. Rather, his objection was that the program had not gone far enough in realizing its potential as "a tremendous social laboratory for research in its field."[68]

The first big disappointment, Weinerman said, was the failure by Weinerman and Dr. J. Paul Fitzgibbon to institute a "personal doctor system" to overcome a major flaw in the program—the lack of doctor-patient intimacy touted as the basic strength of traditional private practice. Failure in this endeavor meant a failure in the major goal to provide good health care to working families, the essence of the program in Weinerman's estimation. The second major flaw, he told the doctors, was board refusal to give members an "active voice" at the highest policy level, the same objection repeatedly raised by the ILWU. In conjunction with this he felt that education and information provided to members was inadequate. These deficits had led to "a halfdraggy feeling of petty grievances and gripes" among Kaiser Permanente patients and staff. As a public health advocate and academically oriented physician, he noticed particularly the "isolation from the community" that resulted from total corporate control, now intensified by Henry Kaiser's personal involvement (Weinerman).

The third program flaw was a lack of board concern, Weinerman believed, for staff welfare and a lack of "true staff autonomy" and "security." The medical staff, he said, must have total and complete control over medical decisions. The most integral part of professional autonomy was direction over personnel policies, and especially the "criteria of professional qualifications." Only by such direction would there be "true internal staff democracy." The loyalty oaths, the threats to Vallejo physicians, and other acts by Kaiser and the trustees, severely undermined the economic and professional security of Permanente doctors. As a member of a group practice system, the physician was unusually dependent on the organization of which he was a part. "We don't have, in a sense, a clientele bound to us personally that is sort of our grip on the economic realities of life," he stated. "We are in a program as doctors *whose patients we don't own*; and if we leave the program we are without anything and we have to start from scratch." Hiring and firing based on corporate loyalty oaths and other whims of the trustees undermined the most basic principles of professional security upon which doctors relied in order to concentrate all their energies on medical practice. This erosion of professional prerogative and autonomy he blamed on the autocratic, "diffuse," and "cumbersome" method of administration (Weinerman).

The issues of professional autonomy and security brought Weinerman's argument full circle back to the loyalty issue. Corporate threats and repression of dissent had drastically interfered with professional practice, an unacceptable turn of events for the medical professionals in the program. He became rambling in his indictment of what had occurred at Kaiser Permanente:

I feel very strongly that racial and political screening policies spell disaster for a nonprofit health program. Basically there is something unAmerican it seems to me . . . about our Government's obligation to control its security and to punish those that are supposed to be treasonous . . . our job is health care . . . not to assume for ourselves the right to decide questions of loyalty . . . based on what the speaker's political position is. Anyone to the left of that being a potential candidate for the disloyalty charge (Weinerman).

"Liberal doctors" were the ones naturally drawn to the Permanente model of group practice, and these would be repulsed by such a requirement for employment. Weinerman called for "decency and courage" in keeping professional boundaries of the program away from the dark political shadows that already hovered over the University of California Medical School. He denied rumors that impugned his own loyalty and integrity that he thought were circulating in the "channels and pathways that seem to go like the wind and over every nook and cranny of the place." He and Kahn were not the only Permanente doctors victimized by the poisoned political atmosphere (Weinerman).

Noting that Weinerman had introduced issues of intense concern, Dr. Irving I. Lomhoff, who was chairing the discussion, remarked that there were more staff doctors present at the meeting than he had ever seen at such an event. Garfield then had the floor. The squeeze Garfield felt between corporate and professional demands resulted in a rare emotional outburst in response to Weinerman. Only through the impressions of others was Garfield's personality usually revealed for the historical record. Rarely did he express his own feelings in public or in writing, and the record of his rejoinder is an unusual revelation of the pressure he now was under. He stammered and rambled in reaction to Weinerman without clear focus. He tried to turn the tables by charging Weinerman with "vagueness" and unsubstantiated accusations that reflected, by implication, on Garfield. He himself had hired "Dick" Weinerman, he said, and it was for him only that Weinerman was working to improve the program. Improvements should be implemented from the executive level downward, not upward from the medical group rank and file. Weinerman was working for him, he reiterated, and not for the "medical service." The only disagreement he had with his "assistant" was on the pace of change, not on the ideals that structured the program (Weinerman).

Garfield sought to dispel the rumor that he thought Weinerman "disloyal to this country." Weinerman had projected several inaccurate ideas through innuendo, he continued. He was sorry if he had "hurt Dick's feelings." But he was forced to clarify Weinerman's position in the organization, and the points of disagreement that now made it impossible for him to stay on as Garfield's hand-picked assistant and possible successor. He stammered that he felt there "is a feeling" that the things Weinerman had mentioned as "ideals for Permanente" were not shared by Garfield. He passionately denied this. He had held these ideals for twenty years, he said, long before he had met Weinerman. And now, he lamented, these beliefs, his integrity, and direction of the program were placed in doubt (Weinerman).

Garfield felt that Weinerman had attempted to divide and conquer, to split the Permanente Medical Group off from administration, to garner support for his own objectives in opposition to Garfield's administration. The issue of "staff autonomy" was brought up, Garfield charged, to suggest that Weinerman was answerable to the medical group, not to Garfield. Weinerman was now his antagonist, "ambitious," easily "frustrated," ready "to step on toes." This was not Garfield's style. He made it clear that Weinerman was hired by him and that he now had the authority to terminate him. Garfield struggled to hold onto his dwindling authority, and the emotional toll was evident in his concluding remarks:

I don't know of any plan in this country that has any more staff autonomy than this. . . . Now if this staff autonomy goes to the point where it means I have to have an assistant that you people want me to have, why, that's basically wrong . . . I insist on the right to pick my own assistant as I would my own wife. And to divorce that assistant as I would my own wife, on my own personal agreement . . . I hope nobody here feels that you have no autonomy because I don't wish a certain person to be my assistant (Weinerman).

Two doctors immediately rose to say that the question of autonomy was not in regard to Garfield's right to choose an assistant, but in reference to professional decisions made by Permanente doctors being "reversed by lay people above and beyond this hospital." A female psychiatrist, new to the staff, spoke from the perspective of her specialty. Dr. Mary Sarvis stated that she had been motivated to work at Permanente rather than elsewhere because of its reputation for individualized quality care. Interference in professional or medical policy by nonprofessional executives and administrators threatened to provoke "an extremely malignant form of helplessness, frustration and resentment" that would cause "grave deterioration of morale and the quality of care." The American Psychiatric Association had stated in the public record that without medical and professional policy control by the medical profession itself, "the quality of practice so deteriorated" that its members were advised against accepting jobs in institutions where this was the case (Weinerman).

That Weinerman was a disruptive and disturbing influence is indicated by the fact that the corporate records do not refer to his brief tenure with the organization, and by the position he accepted immediately upon his departure. He was retained by the AFL-sponsored San Francisco Labor Council to study the feasibility of a union-operated health plan and medical center that would relieve labor's dependence on Kaiser Permanente. He soon published his findings that such a plan was desirable and set about helping to establish one in the Bay Area, though ultimately none materialized.[69]

The conflict between Garfield and Weinerman in 1951 was a symptom rather than a cause of tensions provoked by Kaiser's efforts to assert corporate control over the medical program and by the shortcomings in the Kaiser-Garfield management style. Garfield was able to terminate Weinerman; other opponents were not so easily eliminated. Simultaneous with the Weinerman controversy, Kaiser's high profile and Permanente's controversial philosophy provoked the West Coast county medical societies to fully unleash their hostility against the Permanente doctors.

5 Medical Practice Embattled

The county medical society is the only organization occupying the natural geographic unit and possessed of the necessary professional knowledge and the power to maintain the Principles of Medical Ethics in the organization of medical service in a community.

—AMA report, *Organized Payments of Medical Services*

THE COUNTY AMA AFFILIATES IN CALIFORNIA were the last bulwark of defense against Kaiser's expanding corporate colossus. From 1950 through 1953, county doctors joined in direct battle with the powerful capitalist.

Between 1950 and 1953, at the height of national anticommunist reactionism, aggressive union leaders such as Anthony Anselmo of the Culinary Workers in northern California, Joe DeSilva of the Retail Clerks in southern California, and Harry Bridges had negotiated generous medical benefits for their unions that included employer-paid enrollment in Kaiser Permanente.[1] At the end of 1955 Kaiser membership was well over half a million, less than 5 percent of which were Kaiser employees and their dependents. Organized employee and union groups represented three-fourths of total membership in northern California, the largest region and the site of Kaiser's corporate headquarters. The small nucleus in all regions of 19 full-time doctors who stayed with Permanente after the war grew to more than 500 in the group partnership that developed. They practiced in thirteen Kaiser Foundation Hospitals and thirty outpatient medical centers on the Pacific coast.[2]

In the San Francisco Bay counties, union members and government groups continued to pour into the decentralized Kaiser facilities. The labor affiliation of the prepaid group plan elevated the anxiety level of independent doctors. Although independent urban physicians suffered economic distress as the postwar movement to the suburbs eroded the patient population, hopeful doctors continued to move into the port city. Their numbers increased 30 percent between 1940 and 1950.[3] At the same time massive union support of Kaiser Permanente evoked the specter of socialized medicine. Medical society rejections and verbal attacks on Kaiser escalated sharply in late 1952, climaxing in 1953 and 1954 in both California regions.

In January 1953 the California Medical Association began openly to support the county medical society offensive against Permanente with a scathing rebuttal to an editorial in the liberal *New England Journal of Medicine*. The journal reported that the "Permanente idea" was "worthy of careful study by physicians throughout the country." It represented "one type of program that may not only erect further defenses against the encroachment of socialized medicine, but actually provide more and better medical service, at lower cost, and at the same time maintain the dignity of both doctor and patient." The CMA countered in its journal, *California Medicine,* that "Permanente saved money at the expense of proper patient care" and not only "destroyed" the doctor-patient relationship but also "robbed" the patients of their "freedom" as "captive[s] of the plan." It "bought and sold" members, who were bounced from doctor to doctor. The principal culprit was Henry Kaiser. The editorialist complained, "We have no technical proof that Permanente is the practice of medicine by a layman. But we inevitably end up talking to—or more accurately, being talked to and often threatened by—Mr. Kaiser."[4]

Los Angeles County was the site of Kaiser's greatest expansion, and doctors there perceived Permanente as the destroyer of independent medical practice. LACMA president Dr. Paul D. Foster began a vicious editorial assault in the 5 March 1953 issue of the LACMA *Bulletin,* proclaiming 1953 a year of decision and trial in which the AMA confronted two primary challenges "peculiar" to California physicians. The Kaiser health plan was the first. The second was the entry of labor unions "into the active practice of medicine."[5] Mixing political ideologies Foster warned of corporatism on the right and socialism on the left. Kaiser Permanente and the labor movement were "miniature versions of what state medicine would be were it ever to win out over the free practice of medicine." He noted the ominous "scampering en masse of union members into Permanente."[6]

Henry Kaiser suggested an answer to the attack with a strategy to use the new television medium in a memo entitled "A.M.A. Declares War—The Challenge Is Accepted," dated March 26, 1953. "The labor leaders of the nation will join in taking up the A.M.A. declaration of war," he wrote, "and likewise can take up the fight with the A.M.A. before the American people, because American labor is making it unmistakably known that working people demand better ways to meet the crushing high costs of illness." Kaiser concluded, "Let [the] A.M.A. come face to face with those against whom it has declared war, and let the American people decide for themselves."[7] Kaiser advisers panicked, urging moderation and "dignity" in "accepting the challenge" to public debate, a recommendation in accord with the wishes of the Permanente doctors, who wanted Kaiser to stay out of professional disputes.[8] Apparently Kaiser did not act on the threat to appear on television.

After his advisers had persuaded Kaiser to cool off in deference to the Permanente physicians, in April 1953 Foster issued a proposed resolution to the LACMA Executive Council that echoed a similar resolution by the New York Medical Association against the Health Insurance Plan. The prepaid group plans posed an "inherent threat to the high standards of medical practice, and particularly because of the potential injury to individual captive patients" and "the operation of such closed panel systems in prepaid medical care plans is undesirable and injurious to the public welfare." Thus, "any member of this Association who participates or practices as a member of a closed panel system in a prepaid medical care plan" is acting unethically.[9]

Foster's resolution was part of a nationwide AMA effort to block prepaid group plans. At the June annual meeting in San Francisco, a resolution declared unethical the requirement on the part of a "third party" provider "restricting choice of physician to either individual or group practitioners under contract."[10] This would make it impossible for the prepaid plans to continue operation anywhere in the country.

The LACMA Executive Council accepted the resolutions. When delegates to a CMA conference also approved them, one delegate asked Foster why he did not directly name Permanente. Foster admitted fear of a libel suit. Prepaid group plan representatives at the conference for Ross-Loos, ILGWU, and the Culinary Workers health offices believed that if the attack on Kaiser succeeded, the society would next turn against the smaller plans, which had much less political and economic power than Henry Kaiser. They considered action against the CMA under the antitrust or libel laws and the National Labor Relations Act, or, as a last resort, a personal suit against Foster for remarks in a private meeting observed by a Long Beach Central Labor Council representative.[11]

In June 1954 the AMA House of Delegates meeting in New York proposed to revise the code of medical ethics to state that prepaid, closed-panel medical plans were "unethical." The measure, Resolution 16, was scheduled for presentation to the AMA annual meeting in Florida. Saward, Collen, and other regional leaders took it as a direct assault on Permanente. Ernest Saward was convinced that with the Washington State Supreme Court decision against the King County Medical Association in the Group Health Association of Puget Sound case, Permanente could block the resolution. Garfield, Saward, and Collen flew to Miami to protest the resolution before the AMA meeting, prepared to file a lawsuit if it was adopted. The appointment of the Commission on Medical Care Plans to study the unorthodox plans, chaired by Midwest moderate Dr. Leonard Larson, stymied Resolution 16. It was withdrawn before a vote was taken.[12]

The other prepaid group plans and labor representatives

who banded together in opposition to LACMA and the CMA in 1953 did not enter into litigation with the societies. Remarks in LACMA publications were not libelous. Moreover, the labor unions had not been effective, acting singly, in establishing their own medical programs.

Foster continued his editorial attack against Kaiser in the May 1953 *Bulletin*. "The Time Has Come," he sing-songed in a parody of Lewis Carroll:

> To talk of many things:
> Of corporations and captive patients
>   And free choice of physicians;
> Of interlocking directorates
>   And tax-free, nonprofit organizations;
> Of industrial magnates—and controlled medicine;
>   And why the sea is boiling hot,
>   And whether closed panels have wings.

Foster portrayed the Kaiser Foundation as "monopolistic" and "devouring," destructive of the basic freedom and "divinity" of struggling individualism. Permanente doctors had "succumbed to the lure of corporate medicine." They were "automatons dispensing treatment via directives from some higher source" to patients who were "captives in closed panel systems." He rejected the Kaiser program as any part of "recognized ethical efforts" to provide medical services.[13]

Kaiser's attorney said that the LACMA editorials contained libelous statements but were in the official bulletin of an organization of which Foster was president, making a lawsuit against Foster difficult and lengthy. Nor would it admit Permanente doctors to county medical societies or stop society attempts to thwart Permanente recruitment of new doctors and specialty board certification. The Kaiser Permanente attorneys agreed that the Permanente Medical Group itself was the proper locus for legal decisions regarding these issues. It was improper for Henry Kaiser and his lay trustees to interfere in medical professional affairs.[14]

Simultaneous with medical society rejection of Permanente doctors, a series of antitrust lawsuits filed by prepaid group plans followed the 1943 Group Health Association U.S. Supreme Court precedent in all the West Coast states. The

Group Health Cooperative of Puget Sound was created in 1946. In 1950 Garfield arranged for it to cover 2,000 ILWU members at the port of Seattle, where there was no Kaiser facility. Like GHA, the Puget Sound cooperative depended on outside hospital facilities. As in the GHA case, area hospitals refused to grant staff privileges to Group Health doctors, even in emergencies, and the King County medical society denied them membership. Like their colleagues in other prepaid group plans they thus were unable to gain certification by specialty boards that required society membership. Group Health doctors filed suit under a state constitutional provision that forbade agreements to fix prices or to limit the production of any commodity. On November 15, 1951 the state supreme court found for Group Health. The court strongly condemned the medical society for hindering development of private medical programs.[15]

In March 1952, four months after the Washington court decision, the California superior court ruled in favor of the Complete Service Bureau (CSB) in litigation with the San Diego County Medical Society for its refusal to admit CSB staff physicians into membership. The court upheld the legality of the CSB group plan, which the society had countercharged was engaged in the illegal "corporate practice of medicine." Appeals dragged on until 1954, when the state supreme court upheld the CSB. Even then CSB had to file a $500,000 damage suit before the San Diego County society reinstated four doctors and agreed "to consider" the other doctors "in time."[16]

The Kaiser legal staff followed developments closely. After the state court affirmed the legality of the CSB incorporation, Kaiser attorneys recommended incorporation of the Kaiser Foundation Health Plan, formed in 1946 as a nonprofit trust. The Kaiser trustees managed to stay on firm legal ground throughout the difficult 1940s and 1950s, while the AMA's court losses and expensive campaign against national health insurance from 1943 to 1949 eroded the association's influence in public affairs.[17]

As the Permanente physicians fought for acceptance by their society colleagues, community support of Kaiser Permanente grew rapidly. Foster's attack signified the medical society's powerlessness in the face of Kaiser's expansion in 1953.

On the same day that LACMA approved the Foster resolutions in 1953, the Long Beach *Labor News* endorsed construction of a $16 million city health care facility for lease by the Kaiser Foundation. AFL and CIO unions in the area warned that city-run hospitals "might not be operated to give the working man the best." The unions trusted Kaiser Permanente, but they were suspicious of other providers encumbered by insurance salespeople, insurance company profits, and "inefficient private office operation."[18]

Kaiser was unstoppable. Four months after approval of the Foster resolutions, the Steelworkers' local in northern California at Pittsburg requested the national union to allow Kaiser coverage for its approximately 10,000 members and dependents. Journalists described a "pitched battle" by local AMA physicians to attract workers to their newly devised "Doctor's Plan," called the East Contra Costa County Medical Service. Before the union vote the doctors and their wives camped in the parking lot of the steel plant, swamping workers with leaflets admonishing them over a loudspeaker system to support their "family doctor" by rejecting Permanente. In case they were barred from the plant lot, the doctors planned to drop the leaflets by airplane. Despite these efforts union members voted for Kaiser by a five-to-one margin.[19]

In December 1953 the CMA House of Delegates voted to "notify Congress" of their opposition to all forms of "collectivism." Representatives also announced they were "close to victory" in the first "battle" in "an all-out campaign against the Kaiser Plan." The press reported that 200 doctors in the San Pedro District Medical Society plan organized under the California Physicians' Service "stole a thousand member Culinary Workers' contract right out from under Kaiser's nose"; that 45 percent of the Culinary Workers who were Kaiser members still used private physicians and not the Kaiser plan; and that the 9,000-member International Association of Machinists at the Santa Monica Aircraft Plant turned down Kaiser in favor of the local CPS plan. Added parenthetically was the fact that Sidney Garfield made a salary of $106,000 annually, plus $200,000 from the sale of his "interests" to Kaiser hospitals. Kaiser deflated the CPS triumph by "hailing" it a "victory for the people."[20]

A CPS spokesperson admitted that Kaiser retained the advantage in the labor market. Other AMA county medical society affiliates tried to compete with new plans under CPS. A plan for ILWU Longshoremen in Stockton had long-term success only because Kaiser did not move into the area.[21] Kaiser continued to sign up large groups, such as the cannery workers, even at the peak of the CPS thrust. Long Beach doctors offered coverage as well, but Kaiser's most expensive monthly contract of $12.50 was still $4.50 a month less than their most comprehensive coverage.[22] The fragmented and jerry-built CPS county plans could not compete with Kaiser for union group members.

California labor unions openly defended Kaiser Permanente against the medical society attack of the early 1950s. An AFL health and welfare conference "served notice on the California medical profession . . . that it should re-examine its present policies or face the consequences," more union health centers; in the meantime, the AFL conference strongly endorsed Kaiser: "We conclude that the Kaiser Foundation Plan is at this time the most attractive one to trade union groups." The labor press called the Foster resolutions an unwarranted "sneak attack" on Kaiser. Retail Clerks president Joe DeSilva challenged the societies to engage in an open television debate on the health plan. Southern California unions monitored medical society threats to Kaiser and other prepaid group plans.[23]

As the courts upheld the rights of prepaid group plan doctors against the medical societies, labor and the popular press boosted Kaiser's image. *Look* magazine, the *Saturday Evening Post,* and Chet Huntley of the American Broadcasting Company extolled the health plan as a boon to the American family.[24] Media prophet Norman Vincent Peale was a Kaiser favorite. Peale's formula for material success, "prayerize, picturize, and actualize," was supported by businesspeople, many of whom provided their employees with Peale publications. The dictum that "Christianity has a considerable stake in capitalism" appealed to Kaiser as well. In October 1949 Henry Kaiser gave a sermon before Peale's congregation at Marble Collegiate Church in New York City. Two years later Kaiser and his publicists tried to use Peale's television pulpit to promote the Kaiser health care philosophy nationwide. They planned a Kaiser-sponsored Peale television program emphasizing "how closely bodily ills are tied up with people's emotional, mental and nervous upsets." The participants would be Kaiser, Dr. Herman Kabat, and representatives from the UMW. The Kaiser staff warned against "specifically attacking socialized medicine," as it would constitute a lobbying activity and jeopardize Kaiser Permanente tax exemptions. Apparently the media event was not implemented.[25]

Kaiser moved on to less volatile media efforts that did not highlight controversial aspects of the medical program, such as UMW support. In a *Saturday Evening Post* article by Lester Velie the public relations staff sought to downplay Kaiser's "National Health Plan" and the suggestion that it was a prototype for government or a nationwide doctors' program. At the opening of the Kaiser Foundation Hospital in Los Angeles, Kaiser stressed that "doctors themselves have the opportunity to stop socialization of medicine dead in its tracks" while enjoying "excellent incomes and professional working conditions," if they set aside old antagonisms against corporate medicine and prepaid group practice.[26]

Kaiser publicists stressed parents' gratitude at their happy "birthing" experiences. The original "baby-in-a-drawer" feature in obstetrics at Kaiser hospitals had placed the organization in the vanguard of clinical innovation in the care of newborns and their working-class mothers. It was a variation of rooming-in, a progressive East Coast concept tried most visibly at the Yale University School of Medicine, where a number of Kaiser Permanente pediatricians were trained in the 1940s. Dr. Edith B. Jackson, a graduate of Johns Hopkins and a clinical professor of pediatrics and psychiatry at Yale from the late 1930s to the mid-1950s, pioneered the concept with an experiment in rooming-in at the Grace–New Haven Community Hospital from 1946 to 1952, with two four-bed units. Over 400 observers came to see the facilities and care provided in these units, in which mothers and infants were attended by specialized nurses and pediatric fellows. In the relaxed environment mothers were trained in child care and nurturing. The Kaiser hospitals were unusual in the specific filing-drawer design of their rooming-in units, in the focus on personalized care that reflected values of individualism and assertive behavior in the early bonding and nurturing between mother and baby, and in the extent the concept was implemented.

The Permanente group attracted young idealistic doctors from Yale, among them Alice Friedman and Louise Burr, and there were others attracted from eastern colleges. According to Friedman, they were drawn by "the idea of the thing and the absence of having to bill people and charge for your services." She believed that the caliber of pediatricians attracted to Permanente in the early days was unusually high. Her colleague Alex King came from Johns Hopkins.[27]

In the early 1950s female members of the Kaiser plan and their offspring were thus granted an unusual degree of autonomy and self-determination in the areas of maternity and pediatrics. A member of the Retail Clerks spoke, she said, for many other female workers and workers' wives in thanking Henry Kaiser for "comfort and happiness." This was her fourth child, and she was the only one on the maternity floor with a "planned baby." The low cost of the health plan was a boon to families with unplanned obstetrical expenses. Planners at Fontana gave 40 percent of total bed space at the new hospital to obstetrics, when the California State Bureau of Hospitals recommended 20 percent of total capacity as sufficient. Dr. Raymond Kay assured Garfield that Fontana's fifty to sixty deliveries a month justified the large number of maternity beds.[28]

One historian gives eight reasons that "family-centered" maternity and infant care "did not become the norm" elsewhere in the 1950s and 1960s. The New Haven experiment went against the traditional trends in the medical profession and in institutional care of the period when medical science and authority superseded individual patient needs as goals in hospital administration. Such care entailed "radical revision of the 'hospital-centered' routine" in place since the 1920s, as well as "revolutionary changes in nursing care" (when nurses were finally gaining the professional status they had sought since the 1920s) and in the authority physicians and nurses wielded over parents. Rooming-in rejected the commonly held notion that infants in regular contact with adult family members and visitors would contract and spread infection. It repudiated the traditional child development theory, promulgated by L. Emmett Holt, Sr., in 1920, that "babies under six months old should never be played with" or comforted, else they be "spoiled." Rather, it operated on the revolutionary postwar ideas of Dr. Benjamin Spock that a "child's freedom to learn, and his capacity for self-discipline" were in fact "rooted in his infantile and early childhood *satisfactions.*" On a more material level such experiments in family care did not attract the attention of biotechnology and scientific medicine that hospital administrators and physicians sought to add stature to their institutions. Finally, rooming-in may have appeared to be the incursion of a female folkway into a domain in which male doctors had asserted authority relatively recently. Hospital delivery was not the experience of most women in the United States until the mid-twentieth century. In 1940, 55 percent of U.S. births were in hospitals; by 1950, 88 percent.[29]

Kaiser's "baby-in-a-drawer" version of rooming-in was featured in *Look* magazine articles in 1952 and 1953. In the larger Los Angeles and San Francisco hospitals, "individual nurseries" were behind each bed on the maternity floor. The newborn's stainless steel bassinet could slide like a file drawer back and forth through the wall separating the mother's room from the nursery so that each mother could "slide her baby in beside her own bed when she wants to see or tend it herself." Such personalized pediatric care continued after mother and baby left the hospital. A *Look* photographer followed nine-month-old Patricia Neeland and her mother through Patricia's well-baby check at Oakland Permanente. The article emphasized personal attention by nurses and doctors, and a thorough multiphasic examination.[30]

Kaiser was more interested in representing the health plan as a boon to the average family of the 1950s than in breaking new medical ground in the pediatric and maternity wards. Like *Fortune, Look* was a Luce publication sympathetic to Kaiser. Its writers and editors were most cooperative in allowing

Kaiser staff to preview, edit, and rewrite articles. The Kaiser staff paid particular attention to photographic layout, surmising that "subtle use of pictures" would "dispel criticisms against the plan." "Three of four typical health plan families, fairly photogenic with several kids," were "to serve as models in showing that the plan was aimed strictly at low income and union groups," with at least one family from the University of California faculty. Henry Kaiser, Jr., Garfield, and other doctors and attorneys combed drafts of the articles, amply redlining their contents.

The proofreaders let stand a portrait of Henry Kaiser as the "rugged individualist" who wanted "peace" but was not afraid of the AMA. "If organized medicine wants a fight with Permanente, it will find a worthy foe in the crusty old industrialist," the *Look* reporter asserted. Kaiser's associates warned that "if a fight is forced and anybody doubts the outcome, they point to cement, shipbuilding, steel and aluminum for the answer." He quoted Kaiser, who "rumbled":

There's a revolution going on in medicine; and a lot of doctors still can't see it. People just can't pay for medicine at today's prices. Opposition? Of course some doctors are opposing Permanente. They got all kinds of fool laws passed against the automobile too. But they couldn't keep them from coming. Group medical practice will come too, either that or we'll have socialized medicine, and I think we've got [the term *slipshod* deleted here in red pencil] enough operations going on in Washington now without letting them take over medicine.[31]

Kaiser thus continued to tout the democratic, holistic philosophy integral to preventive health maintenance for patients, while he often assumed a condescending air toward physicians. Politically, he stayed close to the middle road between left-wing laborites who urged socialized medicine and conservative Republicans. The Kaiser health plan record spoke for its economic appeal to working-class families. At the same time, union studies showed that at least 12 percent of the ILWU Warehousemen families who chose indemnity insurance over Kaiser had yearly medical expenses beyond reimbursement as high as 11 percent. Weinerman's study for the

AFL San Francisco Bay area unions showed in 1952 that group prepaid plans nationwide paid an average of 88 to 93 percent of total medical costs, while traditional insurers, including Blue Cross–Blue Shield, covered only 46 to 73 percent. Even though prepaid group plans covered only 3 percent of the population nationally, and only 12 percent in California, by the mid 1950s, Kaiser Permanente covered 65 percent of AFL union members in the twenty-seven labor-management negotiated plans in which it was an option.[32]

Accessibility, economy, and democratic treatment of patients were benefits that offset Henry Kaiser's adamant refusal to grant official union representation in his boardrooms. Pressure by large group subscribers over the years also caused Kaiser Permanente to modify its coverage of treatment for mental illness. Henry Kaiser rejected a request by California's governor, Earl Warren, to serve on the National Association for Mental Health's Commerce and Industry Committee in 1949, despite recognition during the war by union leaders and organized medicine of the special stresses endured by industrial workers. Family dependents complained that Kaiser rejected them on even the slightest evidence of emotional illness. The policy especially affected women. One subscriber claimed that his wife was rejected for membership only because she "had trouble sleeping nights." In a personal letter to Henry Kaiser, another woman protested that though her husband was accepted under a group policy, she was not. This was because she said she had seen a psychiatrist for five months the previous year. She told Kaiser that such action perpetuated a "stigma" against preventive care for mild mental health problems.[33]

Large group enrollments meant that Kaiser had to take employed subscribers who might have mental problems, but not dependents. As their caution toward the "family plan" had indicated, Kaiser officials were conservative in extending services to areas with unknown cost and treatment variables. These variables seemed mostly to affect women and families in the areas of obstetrics, family care, and mental health. Not until 1960 was the huge federal employees' group that joined Kaiser in 1959 successful in adding mental health benefits to coverage.[34]

Labor's support outweighed medical society opposition as the Permanente program thrived, and the UMW and Kabat-Kaiser connection were the springboards for an attempted expansion to a new region far from Kaiser's West Coast enclave. The union had attempted to contract with doctors and hospitals in the Southeast on an individual fee-for-service and per diem basis. After the miners' health fund was created in 1946, five-cent per coal ton royalties paid by consumers provided hospitalization and medical care in hospitals for union members and their dependents. The *Saturday Evening Post* estimated that Lewis took $400 million into the Health and Welfare Fund from coal royalty payments between 1946 and 1952. Yet the money could not buy competent local doctors experienced in group practice and willing to work for a union-controlled plan. Instead, UMW medical director Warren Draper obtained care for miners through an ad hoc system of individual contracts and fee-for-service based on "prevailing community rates." Draper was proud of the "intentional vagueness" of the program and the effect of his influence on organized medicine. State medical societies had named committees "to work out mutual problems," Draper told a magazine reporter. The same reporter praised the program started by another union medical director in 1947 to send miners previously diagnosed as hopeless to rehabilitation centers like Kabat-Kaiser for treatment.[35]

Draper reported to the AMA that from late 1949 through 1951, the fund paid almost $73 million to 6,800 individual physicians and 750 hospitals that regularly participated in the union program, covering 1.5 million potential beneficiaries. However much Draper's system might please the AMA, it failed the miners. "After four years of fiddling and losing money," Kaiser attorney Todd Inch reported in 1951, "they [the union] frankly state they are coming to Permanente because they cannot do the job."[36]

Garfield made an extensive trip to the mining areas and conferred with Draper and Josephine Roche, another union fund trustee. He finally proposed that forty Permanente doctors provide care in Kaiser hospitals located in Beckley, West Virginia, with branches in Logan, West Virginia, Norton, Virginia, and Harlan, Pikesville, and Hazard, Kentucky. The

Welfare Fund would donate $5 million to create a new Kaiser Permanente region. Garfield enthusiastically began recruiting Permanente physicians to implement the ambitious plan in 1951.[37] Draper's optimism about the resolution of difficulties with state medical societies proved unfounded; problems increased rather than diminished. In June 1952 the AMA conducted a highly confidential investigation of the jerry-built UMW medical system. Welfare Fund executives had merely added a new level of bureaucratic complexity to the old contract system that had evolved since the nineteenth century. Home and office care were not covered by the fund but were paid by the traditional check-off system from miners' wages.

Though UMW Health Fund officers obtained a copy of the investigation report, its AMA authors stipulated that no part of it could be released in any form, probably because it would badly damage the reputation of state and county society doctors. The report revealed the prevalence of "unbelievably filthy" facilities operated by unlicensed staff. Services were so "overused" and "abusive" as to be "deplorable." Hospitals were "criminally deficient" in safety and health conditions. Patients were overcharged and neglected. The county medical societies in Kentucky, Tennessee, and West Virginia had little or no communication with union medical officers, and there was no established regulation or complaint procedure. Perhaps organized medicine's efforts to conceal these facts was due partly to the fact that AMA president Elmer Henderson was a Kentuckian. The national association gave the broader ideology of individualism and local control as the reason for resolving problems at the county society level. AMA and local society direction would assure the two "primary principles of free choice of physician by the patient and fee-for-service payment to the physician." "If this program fails with the result that the Fund builds its own hospitals and employs its own physicians," warned the survey team, "then two of the primary principles enunciated by the AMA will be open to question by the public." The report concluded by expressing the apprehension that the miners' fund might decide to build ten of its own hospitals, with two already planned, where salaried physicians would predominate on the professional staff.[38]

The year before the AMA investigation, the Kaiser trustees were deeply involved with reform of the miners' program. Garfield was stimulated by the challenge, but Henry Kaiser was skeptical. He disliked the manner in which the union proposed to reimburse Permanente on a cost-plus basis and the flexibility of a contract "subject to change" at any time by mutual consent. Basically, fund officers would have too much control over affairs to suit Kaiser. He indicated in a discussion with Garfield, Cutting, and Henry Kaiser, Jr., that the UMW stipulation that records of service and costs be open to union officials was unacceptable. Union review, Kaiser explained, "would bring nothing but grief." He added that he did not want the "moral blessings of [the] UMW, but a business-like basis." Yet it must not appear, Kaiser emphasized, that he "declined" to set up UMW hospitals "because we would be associating with John L. Lewis."[39]

The labor leader was entering a decade of declining influence and open antagonism with the UAW's Reuther, whose cooperation was more important to Kaiser. While Reuther enhanced his national prestige as a mainstream spokesperson for labor liberals in the Democratic party, Lewis was increasingly insular and cynical toward the Democratic Left. He withdrew to the inner recesses of what one historian calls his "Kingdom of Coal." But the official reason Kaiser gave for refusing the union was that Garfield and his associates were unable to recruit the additional personnel needed to staff the undertaking. Difficulty in this endeavor and the regional doctor shortage were noted consistently in reports to Kaiser on the proposal. Garfield and Edgar Kaiser continued to express enthusiasm for the project, but the shortage of rural doctors compounded by the inability of Permanente to recruit physicians to go such a distance when the Kaiser Plan in the West was growing so rapidly seemed reason enough to allow the UAW program to fizzle.[40]

The uneasiness of the Kaiser-Lewis relationship was not an admitted cause for the failure of the proposed Kaiser plan. Garfield later said that he introduced them, that Kaiser developed cordial relations with Lewis, and that they became "pretty good friends." But the labor leader probably irritated the industrialist. Garfield admitted that Kaiser did not want to meet Lewis when the miners' health plan first came up but was very sensitive to the possibility of trouble.[41]

Soon Henry Kaiser was in hot water for ill-considered remarks about Lewis at the National Press Club dinner in 1954, where he had announced his intention "to dwell among the people." When asked by reporters what he knew about the "UMW Medical Insurance Plan," Kaiser feigned ignorance except in regard to miners treated at Kabat-Kaiser. Because of their 80 percent recovery rate at the institute, he told the press, Lewis wanted him to set up a complete plan in West Virginia. Kaiser said this invitation was turned down because it would mean overextending Permanente capabilities and detract from the model program already established in the West. Then Lewis "decided that if we didn't do it, he would do it himself," Kaiser said, and surrounded himself with architects and planners to set up his own program.[42]

The UMW fund trustees built ten hospitals in Kentucky, Virginia, and West Virginia under the Miners Memorial Hospital Association, which quickly fell into financial difficulty and ruinous litigation with the state medical societies in Pennsylvania, Ohio, and Colorado. The Pennsylvania society passed a resolution that accused physicians who accepted "payment for their professional services in any other manner than on a fee for service basis" of unethical medical practice. The names of violators would be published semiannually in the society journal. Doctors who engaged in prepaid group practice to treat the miners were denied society membership and hospital privileges in both Pennsylvania and Colorado.[43] Kaiser Permanente endured an identical attack by the West Coast county societies, but its founders had the material resources to build a completely integrated system, and Permanente had a closed-panel physicians' group that practiced only in Kaiser Foundation hospitals. The Mineworkers did not have Kaiser's resources, or the ability to erect facilities near every mining community where it had members. Nor did the union have the ability enjoyed by the ILWU of contracting for care with other viable prepaid group plans able to defend against medical society attacks on the West Coast.

Unfortunately, Kaiser chose this time to declare in the nation's capital, where the UMW had its headquarters, that an organized labor takeover of the medical care system would be more dangerous than "socialized medicine." He elaborated:

There is a danger of medicine being taken out [*sic*] entirely by the labor leaders and then you will not have the competitive aspect that you have under this [Permanente]; and the doctors could be, well, working . . . for the labor leaders of the country and there would be something far more harmful than socialized medicine because it would not be free open competition amongst doctors of this country with their own plans but would rather be plans that are forced upon [them]. And I think this will be forced upon labor leaders if we don't do it.

"I really don't know what his plan is," Kaiser concluded, speaking of Lewis. "I can't answer that question." Reporters assured him that he had given them quite an informative response.[44]

Kaiser's remarks sparked a flurry of activity among his public relations staff. They erased the tape recorded section on Lewis. Kaiser was instructed to "re-record" his answer from a draft prepared for him with the offending phrases "eliminated." But these efforts were too late. The remarks were published in *The Washington Report on Medical Sciences* and passed along to Lewis, Draper, and Roche. A lively exchange of interoffice memos between Roche and Draper expressed glee at the ensuing feud between Kaiser and Lewis. Draper referred to Kaiser's comments as "very fuzzy and confused," but "dastardly." The usually taciturn Roche wrote Draper that she expected he would read Lewis's rejoinder to the industrialist "with great joy."[45]

After informing Kaiser that several UMW representatives had attended the press club luncheon "out of courtesy to you" and confirmed the quotation, Lewis lashed out at Kaiser:

That you of all men should stoop to the utterance of such an unseemly slur leaves me unable to understand your motivation, or to commend your judgment. Perhaps you would like to furnish me with a "Bill of Particulars" in amplification of your blanket indictment. If so, I would be glad to have it. I write this letter conscious of the deeply injurious effect of your statement upon others as well as your own cause.[46]

Draper wrote to Roche of Kaiser: "The perfidy of the man is beyond my comprehension. We have dealt most honorably with Mr. Kaiser" and now "the stature of the individual is indelibly revealed." A week later Kaiser sought to put the dispute to rest with a carefully considered response to Lewis. He conveyed sympathy for labor leaders. He shared their burden, he said, to provide adequate health care for workers and their families because the medical profession itself had failed to provide such care. His statement placed blame for this inadequacy upon the doctors, not organized labor. The physicians were their own worst enemies because they had allowed the medical system to deteriorate to such a critical state that socialized or lay-controlled medicine might result.[47]

Kaiser and his advisers ultimately vetoed expansion to the Lewis stronghold in the Southeast; nor would the Permanente Health Plan extend to Reuther's domain in the near future. It would remain nearer Kaiser's wartime industrial headquarters in the Far West during the magnate's lifetime. Garfield apparently was too distressed and embarrassed to notify Draper of his failure to get final approval for the UMW project from the Kaiser board, having expressed assurance of a favorable decision to him the day before the board's vote. Garfield asked Trefethen to pass along the bad news, which was as much a shock to the UMW trustees as it was to Kaiser's chief medical director. Garfield expressed his sincere regrets to Draper, saying that "the complicating factor of the Stanford University possibilities" were to blame."[48] Henry Kaiser had become fixed on the idea of an affiliation with Stanford to enhance Kaiser Permanente prestige and also to facilitate Permanente recruitment of doctors from the Stanford Medical School.

As late as 1955, reformer Michael Davis in *Medical Care for Tomorrow* reported that the UMW medical program still was operating on an ad hoc localized basis, though it planned to "integrate" medical service and facilities in the same network from West Virginia to Kentucky as discussed with Permanente.[49] Within a decade Lewis withdrew from mainstream politics simultaneously with a dramatic decline in coal production and unemployment for unionized miners. The paternal and enlightened despot of the coal kingdom was powerless to provide his Appalachian mining families with either decent wages or a way out of their deprivation.[50]

Despite the failure of Garfield's initiative with the UMW, other plans successfully fought Permanente's legal battles, and Permanente doctors won their case in the court of public opinion without a long and risky court duel. The legal tide ran decidedly against the societies. By the end of the decade the AMA openly warned its local constituents that society denial of membership to a qualified physician could constitute a restraint of trade under the Sherman Act "if its activities" as an association engaged in a business "adversely affect a business, such as a prepaid medical care plan." Since many societies in the areas where Kaiser operated had themselves entered into "businesses" such as prepaid and fee schedule plans, they were directly subject to the antitrust rulings in the GHA case in 1943, and against the Oregon Medical Society, the King County Medical Society, and the San Diego County Medical Society in the early 1950s.[51]

In addition to labor support and judicial restraint an ironic conservatism in Kaiser corporate philosophy aided medical society acceptance of Kaiser and betrayed the social idealism of some Permanente doctors. In 1954 New York reformers associated with HIP and other prepaid group practice plans on the East Coast asked Garfield to participate in a conference to form "a Federation of all existing group practice health plans and clinics as a basis to fight the opposition of A.M.A. and other opponents." Garfield told Kaiser that "we should *not* be represented" at the proposed conference. "We'd like to have our cake, but eat it too," Garfield admitted. On the one hand,

we certainly would like to have a group of big name leaders and spokesmen for the people take on the A.M.A. when the A.M.A. is damaging our doctors and preventing the people from getting group practice prepayment plans. . . . But on the other hand, we do not want to be identified with a militant organization fighting for the people's interests.[52]

Henry Kaiser and Sidney Garfield did not seek a social revolution. The practical objectives of the Kaiser trustees contrasted sharply with the objectives of those who sought broader reform. The Kaiser board of trustees spoke the same language as mainstream U.S. physicians who opposed socialized medicine.

The last recorded case of county society rejection in northern California would come in March 1954 when the Alameda–Contra Costa County Medical Association (ACCMA) denied a request for transfer of membership from Michigan's Washtenaw County Medical Society for Dr. Clifford H. Keene, Garfield's successor. Keene said that "regardless of my background, my qualifications, my previous activities or plans for the future, I was not acceptable to their organization because I was associated with the Kaiser Foundation medical enterprises." In Michigan he was medical director at the Kaiser Willow Run plant, on the executive council of the Washtenaw County society for seven years, chair of the council for the past two, and a member of the cancer committee for the state society. Michigan society leaders wrote favorable recommendations to their California colleagues to no avail. After his rejection Keene notified the ACCMA that he had begun an appeal at the national level to the AMA, with copies to the ACCMA, the Michigan Medical Society, and Henry J. Kaiser.[53]

External enemies dropped away, but internal problems intensified as a result of Henry Kaiser's provocative conduct and imperious attitude toward doctors. He had transformed the social and economic landscape of the Pacific West, yet at mid-century he stubbornly refused to decentralize management of the large, complex medical enterprise that bore his name. Maintaining authority in the manner of such nineteenth-century magnates as Andrew Carnegie and John D. Rockefeller, and exercising his hospital stewardship with the paternalism of an earlier era, Kaiser and his deputies acted as overseers of all aspects of hospital management, demanding deference from doctors, patients, and staff under their benevolent authority.[54]

Garfield, too, operated in a late nineteenth-century management mode. But he was without Kaiser's aggressiveness, Trefethen's managerial ability, or the business genius of either man. He attempted to manage the fast-growing medical care program as if he were still the country doctor at Desert Center or at Grand Coulee. As long as the medical program remained relatively uncomplicated, he was an effective diplomat between Kaiser and the doctors. His authority was unquestioned by those who began with him at Grand Coulee and the shipyards. He absorbed the hostilities of both sides—the Kaiser trustees and Permanente doctors. With the exponential expansion and stresses of the early 1950s, however, Garfield lost his footing.

In early 1953 Kaiser Permanente facilities included seven hospitals, twelve clinics, one research institute at Belmont, and three rehabilitation centers. The system already provided medical care and hospitalization to approximately 160,000 members in the San Francisco Bay Area, 50,000 in southern California, and 25,000 at Portland-Vancouver. Three new hospitals were under construction in San Francisco, Los Angeles, and Walnut Creek in northern California east of Oakland, near Kaiser's estate at Lafayette. The projected $9.5 million building program for the three new hospitals intensified conflict with the county and state medical societies and precipitated an internal crisis. (See table 5.1.)

When Trefethen confronted Kaiser with Garfield's administrative shortcomings, Kaiser said that he and Garfield had worked hard into the "wee hours" of the morning discussing "various reports" that had come to Trefethen's "ears." Kaiser hoped to find solutions before "the tragedy of the criticisms" harmed the physician.[55]

Probably the "tragedy" was the charge by disaffected physicians in northern California that growing corporate influence had destroyed philosophic principles for which the Permanente doctors had withstood medical society attacks and ostracism. Dr. Weinerman had represented the activist left wing of the physician's group. Raymond Kay in southern California and J. Paul Fitzgibbon in Oakland had openly supported him. Saward and Kahn also shared Weinerman's democratic philosophy, at odds with the corporate conservatism in the Kaiser

TABLE 5.1. Comparison of Kaiser Foundation
and U.S. Hospitals by Beds

Beds	% U.S. Hospitals 1955	Kaiser Foundation Hospitals December 1953	
Under 25	17.3	——	
26–50	25.8	Dragerton, Utah	(30)
		Fontana, Calif.	(35)[a]
51–100	23.1	Walnut Creek, Calif.	(70)[b]
		Richmond, Calif.	(100)[c]
101–200	18.8	——	
201–300	8.1	Los Angeles, Calif.	(210; later 600)[b]
		San Francisco, Calif.	(245)[b]
		Vancouver, Wash.	(250)
		Vallejo, Calif.	(300)[d]
Over 300	6.9	Oakland, Calif.	(310)

SOURCES: Memo, Sherman Adams from Chad Calhoun, ca. end of January 1953, carton 88, HJK Papers; Vallejo *News Chronicle*, 21, 22 March 1947; Northern California Region, *KP Reporter* 10, 5 (June 1967); "Magnitude of Physician Top Management Responsibilities, 6 December 1955, carton 309, HJK Papers. Booklet: "The Inside Story," carton 87:18, EFK Papers. Stevens, *In Sickness and In Wealth*, 230 (table 9.2).
[a]The old hospital at the steel plant was cut into sections and moved to form part of the new facility.
[b]Built in 1953.
[c]Sold to the Permanente Foundation by the U.S. government after World War II for $197,393.
[d]The Permanente Foundation acquired the hospital built for 40,000 new war workers at Mare Island Navy Yard for $221,875 in April 1947, after the city of Vallejo as lessee was unable to sustain it as Vallejo Community Hospital.

boardroom. Ironically in light of the reactionary political environment nationally, medical program leaders appeared to move closest to an extreme liberal position in 1951, with their identification with Bridges and the CIO unions, and with the Weinerman appointment.

During the McCarthy era, Garfield appointed Weinerman to the highest position held by an avowed leftist, despite his brief tenure. Earlier public health ideologues like C.-E. A. Winslow and Henry E. Sigerist viewed medicine's scientific role as secondary to its social mission. A Sigerist disciple,

Weinerman drafted the position paper for the American Public Health Association Subcommittee on Medical Care in 1948. Its members included Isidore Falk and Nathan Sinai. Their recommendation for reform of the national medical system went beyond the CCMC's of sixteen years before, advocating the right to adequate medical care of every U.S. citizen, regardless of the ability to pay. They further advocated federal administration of a public health care system through compulsory insurance and general revenues.[56]

As Kaiser revealed on the national political stage in the 1940s and early 1950s, he strongly opposed socialized medicine and even the milder Wagner-Murray-Dingell bills. Probably neither Kaiser nor Garfield understood the significance of Weinerman's philosophic position when he first arrived in northern California. As a populist Kaiser might have accepted Weinerman's statement that "there must of course always be real democracy . . . through all levels of the program," but certainly not its practical implications. Weinerman sought to bring both doctors and union members into the policy-making process and to establish a "personal physician" system. He vigorously applied public health methods in the multiphasic screening program for the ILWU. Weinerman emphasized the problems of "isolation from the community" and threats to staff and physician "security" posed by corporate interference.[57] He was quickly ousted from Kaiser Permanente.

Cecil Cutting remarked that Henry Kaiser saw the Permanente doctors as employees on the corporate payroll, "like his executives in other industries." Corporate attorney Scott Fleming made the same observation. "Henry Kaiser hoped to control the doctors," he said, "just as he controlled his manufacturing and other operations. The doctors' sense of independence bothered Kaiser."[58]

Kaiser sought to control the doctors by placing Garfield in control of finances, facilities, and equipment purchases. He stated his shock or disbelief that the generous financial arrangements whereby the medical groups received almost 40 percent of monthly health plan dues, with an annual 7 percent bonus if they "fully performed their contractual obligations," did not satisfy them. The $25,000 to $30,000 salaries of top doctors and the average for Permanente partners of $18,500 certainly compared favorably with the earnings of doctors in private practice, averaging about $13,500.[59]

His attitude that the doctors were salaried employees was irritating enough, but Kaiser continued the annoying habit of addressing them in a paternalistic tone when he was in a patient mood, and imperiously when he felt less tolerant. These extremes were so natural for him that he might express both in a single exchange. In May 1953 the magnate summoned all of his elocutionary skills to placate independent local doctors concerned about the new hospital at Walnut Creek. Seeking "sincerely, frankly," and openly "to dispel all sorts of erroneous impressions and rumors," he hoped that they would "join hands" with him in serving "the people" of the community in a competitive spirit. Kaiser's idea of direct involvement with the community at Walnut Creek stopped at the front door of his hospital. "It should be understood," he told the local doctors, "that this is not a community-owned hospital, with funds raised by charity, by the people or government of the community or through federal subsidy." Instead, he declared, "the Walnut Creek Hospital is a Kaiser Foundation Hospital built with funds provided solely by the Foundation itself and it therefore is the responsibility of the Trustees of the Foundation." He refused their request for a proportion of staff positions at the new facility. Since the Kaiser Foundation financed the multimillion-dollar expansion program then underway, the trustees would select the staff, he said, as was the "established pattern" in all Kaiser Permanente regions.[60]

Garfield recognized things that were "a little bit unusual" about Kaiser's intense interest in the Walnut Creek project, and his tendency toward financial extravagance. Soon he saw that Kaiser wanted it to be "the greatest thing he ever built."[61] Garfield recalled:

We were building three hospitals at that time. San Francisco and Los Angeles we kept to a modest amount [of investment]; Walnut Creek Mr. Kaiser got into and he didn't want to abide by any of our rules; and I understood that and went along with it as much as I could. Meanwhile the doctors were getting very mad at me *for* going along with it. . . . The thing that shook us up was that up to that time, he had never interfered with us; he liked what we were doing and stayed out of it. But after he married Ale, he switched all of his interest—it's amazing what love can do—he switched all of his interest into the hospital. That became his key thing; and with his own dynamic way, we couldn't hold him down . . . he didn't want me in the operation at all and I just stayed out of it.[62]

Family and medical affairs became enmeshed. After his own marriage in early 1951, Kaiser encouraged Garfield to marry Ale's sister Helen, also a divorced nurse. The newlywed Kaisers thought she would make an excellent spouse for the young, debonair, and long-divorced Sidney Garfield. The second marriages of the two men made them brothers-in-law and next door neighbors, as the Garfields moved adjacent to the Kaisers. Clifford Keene recalled that the proximity and constant contact of the two couples provoked "the most horrendous fights, embarrassing arguments and explosions" between the men, which Garfield customarily lost. Afterward Kaiser was remorseful. Nightly cocktail hours became an intimate family ritual, associates believed, at which the Garfields and Kaisers decided critical issues about the medical program. Because of "that peculiar relationship," Clifford Keene later noted, "a nice definition of organizational pattern" separating medical, professional, and business aspects of the program was "impossible." This blurring of the lines of authority continued for several years.

The Walnut Creek hospital was the progeny of the marriages. Rumors flew that Alyce Kaiser was not yet accepted as part of the "executive family" and saw control over the new hospital as an opportunity to establish herself. Garfield and Trefethen both supported the Kaisers in the Walnut Creek plan, despite the paucity of Kaiser Plan members in the area, and the danger that the program was expanding too fast for the funds on hand.[63] Permanente doctors reacted vehemently against the new hospital. Alyce Kaiser, not they, chose Wallace Cook as the medical director; Alyce Kaiser, not they, handpicked the rest of the staff without consultation and assumed the role of chief administrator. Henry Kaiser visited the facility daily and ordered for it the latest and most expensive building material and equipment. It was a one-story, ranch-style design "in an outdoor country atmosphere: with land-scaped lanais that patients could enter from their rooms through full-view sliding glass doors. Individual electric beds were equipped with hot and cold running water, ice water, radio, nurse's call, and floor to ceiling draw curtains for privacy.[64]

The financial strain soon was evident even to the "not very frugal" Kaiser. By the time Walnut Creek opened, the Kaiser Foundation reported large deficits that threatened to delay completion of Los Angeles and San Francisco facilities for which the doctors felt they had sacrificed income.[65] Complaints about deteriorating quality rose, especially in San Francisco.

Corporate accounting projected a $440,000 cost overrun in the Northern California Division as a result of construction and remodeling. Garfield also had to confront financial problems in southern California within the medical group. The southern group required an additional $10,000 a month income to offset its deficit by the end of 1953. A $1.00 per member a month increase in dues instituted by Kay stirred Kaiser's anger because he was not consulted. Kaiser was "shocked" at discovering this unauthorized action. Keeping tabs on hospital and health plan budgets became an obsession, and he frequently expressed "shock," "dismay," and "amazement" at the inefficiencies of his subordinates.[66] He was particularly irritated by physicians' complaints over the allocation of his financial resources.

Kaiser was even less tolerant of the Permanente doctors than he was of their medical society opponents. Because he controlled the finances, he was confident of winning any dispute, always reducing professional issues to the matter of the doctors' financial dependence. The month Walnut Creek was to open, and on the long night he spent with Garfield into the "wee hours" instructing him to withdraw from medical group affairs, Kaiser wrote a rambling memo to group doctors. He threatened to punish them for their complaints about Walnut Creek, refusing to purchase their equipment. "Dr. Garfield definitely has decided," Kaiser wrote the rebellious physicians, "that he must cease trying to help the Medical Groups because the help he has sought to give has been misunderstood as control of the doctors." He continued, speaking of himself in the third person. "Since Henry Kaiser has repeatedly stated that neither he nor the other Foundation Trustees are in any way entering into the medical groups' operations, Mr. Kaiser feels that it has been a mistake for the Kaiser Foundation to finance the medical groups' equipment, facilities and improvements." The message was clear: removal of corporate financial aid was the price of physician "autonomy" and control over the practice of medicine inside Kaiser hospital walls.[67]

Permanente doctors were more distressed by Kaiser's autocracy than by his financial power. He failed to gauge the depth of their increasing resentment. He did not recognize the strength of the leadership and group solidarity that emerged as Garfield's influence waned. Now Kaiser set out to challenge this powerful group consciousness. He proposed a new organization, breaking up the large regional groups into smaller partnerships. A separate group at Walnut Creek would give Henry and Alyce Kaiser sole control. "Competition is the very essence of the American system," Kaiser lectured the doctors at Walnut Creek in 1953.[68]

Oakland medical director Morris Collen recalled that Mrs. Kaiser "handpicked" the best doctors from Oakland for the "ideal medical center" she envisioned at Walnut Creek. Henry and Ale Kaiser "wanted to disassociate Walnut Creek from the medical group, set their own salaries, and set up a separate partnership," said Collen. Ale Kaiser "wanted to run it completely autonomously . . . outside of the rules and policies of the Permanente Medical Group." "Oakland would be separate; San Francisco would be separate; Walnut Creek would be separate. This divide-and-conquer approach was very clear," said Collen. The Kaiser board "then would control everybody because they already controlled the members."[69]

Garfield supported the idea of smaller groups on differing salary scales as compatible with the competitive principle. But Trefethen admitted that the plan was the result of Kaiser's "pique" at the doctors rather than of an organizational philosophy. He observed that "Henry just felt that these doctors were getting too big for their britches." Breaking them into smaller units would make them more manageable. In this case Trefethen and other management executives supported the Permanente physicians. "Some of the rest of us felt," Trefethen states, "that we were strong enough to handle them. We believed in area competition, but we didn't believe in competition within an area, and so we prevailed in that. . . . We couldn't even figure out how to administer it."[70]

Trefethen now saw a sharp break develop between Garfield and Kaiser. Kaiser "became very critical of Sidney, and Sidney was critical of him," Trefethen said. "Henry wouldn't even speak to Garfield for a while."[71] Garfield was caught between Kaiser and the doctors in the allocation of tight resources. They "got very mad" at Kaiser's extravagance at Walnut Creek, Garfield recalled. "They felt that I was letting them down. . . . We had to hold San Francisco down to minimum expenditures for equipment, for everything, while Walnut Creek seemed to be spending a great deal of money . . . they thought it was unfair, and they realized I couldn't protect them from it." Then Kaiser was angry at Garfield because he could not win the doctors over to his side.[72] Trouble escalated.

The mild-natured Garfield could please no one. He was caught in the crossfire between the AMA county societies and the Permanente doctors, and now between Kaiser and the doctors. Henry Kaiser conveyed his dissatisfaction via copious memoranda regarding Garfield's management blunders. He blamed the medical group for all the headaches thrust upon the trustees. He told Garfield to give the Permanente doctors all responsibility for purchases to remedy their complaint that the leasing and equipping of the medical facilities did not represent "corporate control."[73]

Kaiser failed in his efforts to dilute group strength. The Permanente executive committee drafted a lengthy report to Henry Kaiser refusing the separate partnership plan. Wally Cook, selected to head the Walnut Creek group, agreed. Collen presented the refusal to Kaiser at his Lafayette home. Kaiser "threw it on the coffee table" demanding to know the meaning of "all this gobbledy-gook." He stormed angrily out of the room without reading the full report from the dissenting doctors.[74]

Kaiser spent several months in the fall of 1953 chiding Garfield for his failures in expediting facilities construction, while Kaiser's own actions continued to fuel discontent within the medical group. Factionalism in the northern California medical group had resulted in a rash of leave-takings and resignations by top doctors. Fitzgibbon had left in June, Cutting believed, because he feared the growing corporate influence. He had told Cutting, "We're going to be dominated by the Kaiser people and it'll be another staff employed physician kind of arrangement." In mid-October LaMonte Baritell, medical director at Oakland, resigned "suddenly and unexpectedly." Garfield held a special meeting with the medical group to discuss Baritell's complaints, which centered on financial differences with the corporate trustees. Baritell thought that Garfield's frugality and refusal to buy equipment and to hire more doctors and nurses threatened program survival. Perhaps frugality appeared conspiratorial in light of Kaiser's extravagances at Walnut Creek. Collen also was disgruntled, not only at Garfield but at Baritell as well. Baritell objected to his Medical Methods Research activities. He too helped spin the web of growing discontent.[75]

Kaiser believed that the main problem was Garfield's inability to delegate responsibility. Matters he was accustomed to handling on a personal basis, especially relations with the medical groups, became too unwieldy with program growth for Garfield's personal management. He continued to rely only upon old associates, such as Cutting and Neighbor, with him during the simpler days at Grand Coulee. Kaiser tried to help him restructure his administration so that the medical groups would assume more responsibility and develop their own leadership. He suggested creating more departments under a decentralized bureaucracy. "The good the criticisms have done," wrote Kaiser, "is that it has made Dr. Garfield realize that he no longer [can] do the work personally for those who should be delegated to carry the responsibilities." In a companion memo to Garfield, Kaiser seemed most irritated

that Garfield had "constantly tried to help others in the organizations, and this has been misinterpreted—not only by
others, but by me." Kaiser referred to Garfield's continuing
personal involvement with the medical groups. He saw Garfield's divided loyalties and wanted the doctor's primary tie to
be to himself.[76]

Kaiser's efforts to bolster Garfield's authority and to teach
him the proper delegation of responsibility came too late. He
abruptly switched to a more drastic solution, sought by Trefethen and Edgar Kaiser—bringing in Clifford Keene.

6   The Doctors' Revolt and Kaiser's Hawaiian Retreat

Kaiser was so "disturbed" by the situation over Walnut Creek that "he wanted to move me out of the way," Garfield admitted. "The next thing I knew, Gene [Trefethen] asked me if I could take Cliff [Keene] on as my assistant." Permanente leaders viewed Keene's appointment as an attempt to impose firmer corporate control rather than support the democracy of which Weinerman had spoken. Kay remarked bluntly that "Keene was an army colonel and acted like one."[1]

Keene was medical director at the Kaiser-Frazer plant at Willow Run, Michigan. In the summer of 1953, the plant began to fail. Hundreds and then thousands of workers were laid off. Keene began to look for another job. He had an impeccable professional record, strong expertise in industrial medicine, and experience in dealing with the big unions gained through working with the United Auto Workers at Kaiser-Frazer. In addition to his seven years of experience in industry, Keene had a distinguished tenure at the University of Michigan Medical School, both as a student and teacher; as a lieutenant colonel he had served in World War II in the southern Pacific and at large military installations stateside. He was a member in good standing in the local medical societies, in which he held important committee and board positions. Working with Edgar Kaiser, Keene developed a healthy respect for labor economists and union leaders, as well as expertise in negotiation and designing medical programs to meet the needs of their members.[2]

Seven years earlier, after his discharge from the army, Keene with a wife and three daughters was insecure about his future. On his way back to Michigan, with stops in Hawaii and California, he had appeared early one morning on the steps of the old Permanente Hospital in Oakland where Garfield found him in a rumpled uniform, cap in hand. Garfield accepted him for a ten-week assignment in Oakland even though Keene did not have a license to practice in the state, an assignment that provoked the 1946 ethics charge against Garfield. The following month Keene passed the state exams before a hostile state medical board. The Kaiser company then asked him to set up a medical office at Willow Run. In April 1946 Keene reported for duty, believing the controversy in California was an isolated incident in the past.[3]

Now, in 1953, Keene was convinced that his job would terminate when the plant closed. He turned to Edgar Kaiser, whom he regarded highly, for a recommendation to U.S. Steel. He was dismayed by his reception in the younger Kaiser's office. Probably distraught by his own position as overseer of one of Kaiser's only failures, Edgar Kaiser greeted Keene gruffly. Pacing back and forth with a cigarette in his mouth, impatiently jingling the keys in his pocket, he refused Keene's request. "I'm not going to do a damn thing!" he told the doctor when asked to write the recommendation. "You go back to work." Keene was "flabbergasted." He told his wife he was "thrown out" of the office. Shortly he received an even more enigmatic and insulting message for him and his wife to appear at seven o'clock that evening at the Edgar Kaiser home for dinner with Henry Kaiser, who had arrived unexpectedly from Oakland. When the Keenes entered the "small, twenty-four room" Kaiser domicile, they were given only time to tender their cocktail orders before Henry Kaiser launched into a two-and-a-half hour monologue about his relationship with Garfield. "The old man started the conversation," Keene recalled, "with his usual assumption that you knew what he was talking about . . . no preamble, no introduction." Keene had no prior knowledge of either the relationship or the problems between the two men. Occasionally, he had heard of events in California, with no notion that they would effect on his own life. Suddenly his hosts began to bombard him with "intimate and gruesome detail" about Kaiser's problems with Garfield. For several hours after he sat down with the Kaisers, the only comments Keene made were: "I'll have a scotch and water," and "Please pass the pepper."[4]

Henry Kaiser launched into a diatribe. "Sidney wasn't a good businessman, and he wasn't an organizer and he was inconsistent and Mr. Kaiser couldn't understand his business attitude, and neither could any of the other businessmen," Keene quoted Kaiser. "Sidney had handled them so poorly" that the Permanente doctors were "all in rebellion," with Monte Baritell, the medical director at Oakland Permanente, and Wallace Neighbor spearheading the revolt. The doctors were so upset, Kaiser told Keene, that "they didn't know whether they could ever get the thing back together again. On top of it all, the medical societies were out after Sidney and out after Mr. Kaiser, thinking that what they were trying to do was socialism, if not communism." Keene said that Kaiser continued the "harangue" as a "monologue, not a dialogue," until 10:30 or 11:00. Edgar "would chime in," with Sue Kaiser also participating. They complained "about how Sidney did something or other at the dams or in wherever, which they couldn't understand," and he was not good at handling money. Keene extricated himself with the excuse he had to operate the next morning. He asked Henry Kaiser: "What's all this got to do with me?" He "looked at me as if I were an idiot child," Keene continued, and said: "What I'm trying to tell you is that . . . you wouldn't like United States Steel. They aren't our kind of people. . . . I want you to come out there to the West Coast and run this thing." Keene asked Kaiser what he meant. "Put together a medical program and make it go," Kaiser retorted. "We need some business principles."[5]

Keene had an unpleasant trip to Oakland. Henry Kaiser, accustomed to having his own way, hounded him day and night. "I was something he was gonna cultivate," Keene said, "and he *did* . . . the telephone would ring incessantly." Kaiser wanted to know every detail of Keene's movements and feelings, what he said, what he ate, and when he slept. Keene recognized immediately that the degree of the internal professional rebellion against corporate management was critical. His arrival provoked even more hostility. The doctors turned against him as Kaiser's "hired gun." Although corporate friends warned Keene of the rebellion among the doctors and said he would get "his ass kicked off" if he went to Oakland, he was unprepared for the hatred and anger he encountered. "I had never seen such hostile people," he declared. "I have never felt such a venomous attitude toward me in my whole forty-three years of life as was expressed by Ray Kay and Morris Collen." They were incensed "that I should have the temerity or the audacity or the arrogance to come out and think I could . . . be involved in that medical program and do anything about it." The Permanente doctors "practically spit on me!" Keene recalled. He realized he would be "crazy" to accept Kaiser's offer. He called and told his wife they were taking the U.S. Steel position.[6]

The day before he was scheduled to return home, Keene accepted a request by Garfield to attend a private breakfast meeting just between the two doctors. On the morning of December 5 he met Garfield in the Tartan Room at the Mark Hopkins Hotel in San Francisco, bedecked with its somber Highland plaids and medieval military weapons. Garfield ate his "usual" grapefruit with a cherry on top and eggs Benedict while Keene, who had lost his appetite, pushed his own food around his plate.[7]

The breakfast meeting, though "quiet and stilted," was the most momentous event of Keene's stay in Oakland. Garfield's silence prompted Keene to begin. He observed that the medical program was "in a helleva mess," that he would not know how to solve all the problems, and it was Garfield's "baby" to rescue. Garfield put down his grapefruit spoon and made an amazing admission. "Well, the big problem there is that Mr. Henry Kaiser doesn't have any confidence in my ability to manage a program, and everyone agrees the program needs some kind of leadership, strong leadership, and strong leadership hasn't emerged," Keene quoted Garfield. He then asked Keene to come in and see if he could "turn it around."[8] Garfield's direct request changed Keene's mind, though Garfield never later acknowledged making these comments.

Not until fifteen years later did Keene realize that Henry Kaiser forced Garfield to make the dramatic request at the Mark Hopkins. "I'm sure the old man made Sidney do it," he said later. Just the same he was certain he had understood the conditions of his new employment correctly. Kaiser asked him to assume Garfield's position as chief medical director, not as Garfield's assistant. It "made me madder than hell," Keene said. "I've never been anybody's assistant."[9]

Thirty years later, Garfield still said that Kaiser had brought Keene in as his assistant, in the same role as Dr. E. Richard Weinerman two years before. "I agreed to take him on as my assistant," Garfield said. "I think he [Kaiser] wanted to bring him in my place, but the doctors raised so much fuss about it . . . Gene [Trefethen] promised the doctors they would never put him in charge without their approval."

The trustees never clarified what they expected to happen between Garfield and Keene. There was no clearcut transfer of authority. No one in the Kaiser boardroom wanted to escalate internal tensions by designating who, in fact, was corporate medical chief. The Permanente doctors, on the other hand, were concerned that Garfield's poor business judgment threatened their own status in the organization. Most were not long-term Garfield disciples like Cutting, Kay, and Neighbor, and they did not come to his defense as he expected. Kaiser had not recognized either Garfield's organizational shortcomings or the havoc wrought by muddled lines of communication and authority between the corporate and medical branches of the program.[10]

Keene thought that Kaiser treated Garfield in public in a "mean" way. After Keene accepted Kaiser's offer, the industrialist also showed insensitivity toward Dr. Keene. If Garfield had, on occasion, "lied" outright to Kaiser when it was expedient, as close observers charged, Kaiser committed that offense himself.[11]

Kaiser now put all of his energies into easing the pain of Garfield's removal from the top position, while he left Keene to fend for himself. Once Keene came to Oakland, Kaiser turned his full attention to publicizing Garfield's new role as director of facilities construction and geographic expansion, a role Kaiser viewed as more important than day-to-day management.

On the day before Garfield's breakfast meeting with Keene, Kaiser's office drafted a statement making Garfield's fall from authority appear to be a promotion. The Kaiser Foundation had long held the "ambition" to relieve Garfield of daily problems and time-consuming details to free him for work of "greater nation-wide significance" in policy making and expansion of the Permanente concept on a national scale. Garfield would be an ambassador to help start new programs in other parts of the country. He also would oversee relations in the nation's capital, lobbying for legislation to support prepaid group practice.[12]

Prior to this statement on December 4, 1953, there is no evidence that Kaiser approached Garfield about his intentions for Clifford Keene, though such conversations could have been informal. Not until the last two days of Keene's visit to Oakland did Kaiser directly ask Garfield to recruit him "to fill the position which you have developed in the course of the expansion of better medical care" and which it had been "constantly recognized" over the past year someone else must fill. The industrialist applied heavier pressure in a letter dated December 5. "You stated to me recently when I discussed with you what Keene might be offered, that he should be offered such a position," Kaiser claimed. Now he clearly expected Garfield to make Keene and others who "might be upset" by the change accept Keene's appointment. Kaiser placed the responsibility for any ill effects of his decision, already made, squarely on Garfield. "Personally, I am certain there could be no great harm if you would give him every assistance possible to make him a success. . . . There could be harm only if you are unwilling to indoctrinate another individual into the day to day detail work that you have been doing in the area." "Certain of your associates," he continued, "have said that it is unfair to the entire organization to place the whole organization in the position where if something happened to you by accident that no one had been prepared to assume your duties. It is generally conceded that it is not good business in any organization to fail to develop men who can be advanced." He concluded that he wanted Garfield to "become a national figure in the development of better medical care for more people at a lower cost." He attached an outline of what Garfield should be doing "outside of the local area."[13]

Within a week the Kaiser Foundation announced Keene's appointment as "assistant to Dr. Sidney R. Garfield." Keene's official title and function were ambiguous, but a flurry of long-distance calls and teletypes between Oakland and the Keene's Midwest address clarified one fact. Dr. Keene's title was "Executive Associate." He refused to follow in Weinerman's unsuccessful role as "assistant" to the venerable Garfield. The starting salary of $40,000, when Permanente partners averaged only about half of that, indicated the powerful expectations behind the closed door of the Kaiser boardroom. The trustees announced the appointment with little fanfare in the same release that noted Dr. Baritell's resignation as medical director and chief of surgery at Oakland Permanente Hospital.[14]

The two events were simultaneous with the opening of the new San Francisco hospital. They marked the organization's entry into an era of dramatic conflict and change. An omen even darker than Baritell's resignation and Garfield's shifting role was buried in a Kaiser letter to Collen six days later. Kaiser notified Collen of Keene's position as executive associate "to direct Foundation Health Plan and Hospital operation in Northern California." He then chastised Collen as chair of the Permanente executive committee for problems with the medical group. Dan Brown, the group's lay representative, had threatened the corporate attorney George Link that the group "could blow up the organization." Kaiser charged this was an effort to destroy group morale.[15] The medical program moved closer to the brink of disaster after Keene's permanent arrival on the West Coast. Keene described it as "bogged down in personal prerogative, in challenges between personalities, strong personalities . . . in a myriad of suspicions and in a quagmire of antipathies."[16]

A consumer report by a liberal journalist, distrusted by Kaiser officials, laid out the benefits and drawbacks for doctors in the Permanente medical groups. His conclusions were unexpectedly positive: the benefits of group practice in an economically successful system outweighed the negative aspects of collegial ostracism and corporate interference in medical practice. Doctors complained most frequently about patient "overload" and heavy appointment schedules. Patients were dissatisfied with the failure of the "family doctor" system advocated by Weinerman and his supporters. Though the patient could request a certain physician, that doctor might often be busy and a long wait for an appointment the result. In general, however, patients and doctors both were "satisfied" with Permanente group practice. The report summarized the attractive features for doctors. They "felt grateful at being able to devote their full working time to the treatment of patients, with no time lost in the burdensome duties of sending and collecting bills, buying equipment, or other non-medical matters." They liked the "stimulation of working in teams," and referring patients for needed treatment without worrying about "economic barriers." They liked their own "more stable family life" as a result of regular working hours, carefree vacation time, and weekends off.[17]

There were other reasons that Cutting, Saward, and Kay never indicated they had recruitment problems, despite the physician shortage in the 1950s. The prepaid group plan attracted an unusual percentage of women—over 2.5 times the percentage represented in the profession as a whole. In 1955 the Northern California Permanente Group was 14.76 percent female (of 237 physicians, 34 were women), when only 5.5 percent of U.S. medical students were women.[18] Women in medicine felt the responsibilities of nurture and care of their own families, in addition to taking on the nontraditional professional role. They frequently compromised their own careers to sustain their nuclear families with their unpaid domestic service and allegiance to the ideal of domestic tranquility. One female Permanente pediatrician, a specialty most consistent with women's self-perceived nurturing role, described the emotional domestic burden. Like the controversial Dr. Weinerman, Dr. Alice Friedman came west from Yale University, attracted by prepaid group practice. Despite new progressive attitudes in medicine, she was traditional. Though childless, she was a nurturer of children; though of equal professional status with her first husband, Dr. David de Kruif, and her second husband, a Kaiser engineer, she ultimately chose less than full-time employment so that she could devote time to sustaining her household and her marriage. Medical director Wallace Cook, whom Friedman describes as not sympathetic to women physicians, thus asked her to resign as a partner. Friedman continued as a part-time pediatrician at Walnut Creek from 1955 to 1967.[19]

In southern California Raymond Kay emphasized the advantages of group practice to physicians who wanted to spend time with their families. He regarded the bread-and-butter benefits of group practice as essential in recruiting and retaining high quality physicians. These included financial security, relief from business responsibilities with a full focus on medical practice, predictable scheduling that enhanced family life and mental outlook, and "fringe benefits" such as medical and life insurance and a pension plan.[20] Yet Kay expected new recruits to demonstrate philosophic commitment to prepaid group practice beyond the material benefits. "We chose outstanding physicians as our [recruitment] representatives, doctors who combined professional excellence with deep convictions about our Group's objectives."[21]

The consumer report on the health plan pinpointed the doctors' frustrations and discontent, consequences of the domineering attitude and unilateral decision making of the Kaiser trustees. "The fact that the Kaiser health plan is tightly controlled by a board consisting mainly of Henry Kaiser and executives of his industrial empire, without broad community representation, has been sharply criticized," the author noted. Moreover, "funds from the health plan income in one geographic area are frequently diverted to develop facilities in another, rather than used to improve services in the area contributing the 'surplus'." Kaisers expand into new areas "before the quality of medical care reaches sufficiently high levels in the old ones," a clear reference to discontent over Walnut Creek.[22] Conversely corporate officials blamed the quarter of a million dollar deficits by early 1956 on "soaring expenditures by the Medical Group."[23]

The doctors continued to blame Kaiser's extravagance at Walnut Creek for the losses. Open corporate-professional warfare erupted in northern California in the spring of 1955. The resignation of Dr. Paul Fitzgibbon (a founding medical group partner and its regional medical director from 1946–52) in June 1953, and of Dr. A. LaMonte Baritell in October after the flare-up over Walnut Creek, were early dramatic signs of the depth of professional ill will. Baritell was director of research and chief surgeon for the Kaiser Bay Area hospitals, medical director of the Oakland Permanente Hospital, senior partner and executive director of the Permanente Medical Group, and member of the Permanente Executive Committee. The seasoned Cecil Cutting stepped into Baritell's roles as medical director and chief surgeon at Oakland. Four months later Cutting and Collen persuaded Baritell to return. In February 1954 he was reinstated to all of his former positions.[24]

Neighbor and Collen continued to support Garfield. Keene called Neighbor the "ringleader" in the rebellion against Keene's appointment. Cutting was a neutral compromiser, while it is likely that Baritell led the movement to detach further from Garfield during 1954 and into 1955.[25] Baritell and Collen had deep-seated philosophic differences. Collen provided aggressive leadership in preventive medicine and the multiphasic screening program, and Baritell adamantly opposed the preventive medicine programs as economically inefficient, attempting to stop Collen's multiphasic program at Oakland. Collen received Cutting's and Garfield's unwavering support. Baritell's failed coup resulted in his early retirement, but not until 1966, when he opened a vineyard.[26]

At first, northern California stood alone in the revolt against the trustees. Like Kay in the south, Saward in Oregon gained independence from the Oakland trustees, but for an opposite reason. Kay supported Garfield's administration,

Saward did not. According to Saward, Garfield was in the Portland-Vancouver area only four times between 1945 and 1950. He recognized that Saward was the dominant force behind the medical program there, determined to maintain the self-sufficiency and independence that geographic isolation fostered in the region. According to Saward, Garfield considered him an "apostate" because of his formation in 1948 of the Permanente Clinic, independent of corporate control. A separate contract guaranteed the group a fixed percentage of health plan dues to provide hospital and outpatient medical services. Supported by Neighbor, Garfield opposed Saward's move toward independence. Saward later said his independence was seen as an act of "disloyalty" and even of "patricide" against Garfield as "founding father." Nevertheless, the strong director of the Northern Permanente organization prevailed. Never again did Garfield venture into Saward's domain. Now Saward viewed the discontent in northern California with "dispassion." He thought that the northern California program was in trouble because Garfield still perceived himself as "sole proprietor." Garfield had so much emotional investment in his leadership of the medical groups that he refused to let it go even as the warring factions threatened to destroy program integrity, and reorganization became a critical necessity.[27]

A series of Oakland meetings in the early months of 1955 created a high pitch of "bitterness and increased polarization."[28] Kaiser's response to the first signs of rebellion was simple and direct. He responded paternally in a memorandum dated March 1955. "Recently, the attention of the Board has been called to the broad problem of what is termed 'personal security' of the individual physician and the 'security of the group' in which he works," he began, with a condescending reference to complex ideological issues. Rumors and discontent were the result of two factors. The first was "a lack of correct knowledge" by the physicians of the "organization and reasons for being of the various entities which comprise the Kaiser Plan for health care." The second factor also was due to physician misconception. The "inadequacy of communication between the physicians and the various controlling boards" had made it impossible for the boards "to obtain accurate information" about physician problems. This had resulted in responses that were only "temporarily expedient," and that continued to invoke "friction and crisis." The solutions were simple. Kaiser would educate the doctors by a series of letters and meetings in the concepts of a charitable trust and nonprofit corporation. Reorganization would jeopardize their tax-exempt status. Kaiser announced a survey of physician attitudes to quantify the doctors' complaints in an effort to resolve them.[29]

As Kaiser commenced his letter-writing campaign and attitude survey, the doctors showed that their complaints were not just petty grievances due to "miscommunication." They were grounded in a carefully articulated concept of the proper relationship between themselves and the Kaiser trustees. The rebellion was not a simple skirmish resulting from rumor and misinformation as Kaiser suggested. The doctors conceived the entire program as their creation and prerogative; Kaiser saw it as his.

The medical group responded contentiously with a "Bill of Rights" in an April memorandum to Trefethen that echoed the tone of aggressive unionism found among some health plan members. The physicians called for "a mutually satisfactory integration of all management activities, mutually satisfactory representation at policy making levels, mutually satisfactory methods of monetary distribution and control, and mutually satisfactory methods of selection of all key personnel." They concluded: "In the belief that this difference can be resolved through better understanding we request the formation of a Working Council."[30]

The northern California physician leaders formed the Working Council. They were joined by Kay and Saward, to formulate medical group policy and negotiate with the Kaiser trustees. The doctors wanted to control member selection and health plan dues as well as medical services. At its first meeting the council issued a lengthy memorandum informing Edgar Kaiser, Trefethen, Garfield, Keene, and attorney George Link of their escalating demands. Kaiser himself did not attend meetings of the Working Council "because of the urgency of other matters."[31]

The memorandum spelled out every aspect of physician complaint. Garfield, not Kaiser, started the shipyard plan in 1942, as Sidney R. Garfield and Associates. During the war years and during reconversion, up to 1948, "we were completely one team." They continued: "There was never any question but that we were participating in the physician operation of a medical care plan including all of its parts—direct operation of hospitals, direct management of clinics, and direct agreements with the patient membership. Kaiser sponsorship gave us the backing and security we needed to do the job." In 1948 the physicians formed a partnership to supplant Garfield's sole proprietorship. This again was by their own initiative. At the same time a nonprofit hospital organization "was created"—they did not say by whom—in order "to convert a maximum amount of our funds to the construction of facilities for our workshops." Finally, because of problems with the medical societies, and "contrary to the desire both of the trustees and of the doctors, it became expedient to change the direct relationship between the doctors and their patient members by setting up an intervening third party in the form of the Health Plan Trust."[32]

Nevertheless, the "basic concept" of integrated operation of all medical care entities under "physician management" was sustained from 1948 through 1952, when a radical change occurred. "Beginning in 1952," they wrote, "there became apparent a change in the attitude of our trustees which manifested itself in several ways." These they enumerated:

1. The change in the attitude of the Board of Trustees toward its representative, Dr. Garfield.
2. The board, in good faith we are sure, began to enter directly into management.
3. A series of unilateral actions by the board took place, and for the first time lay domination became a matter of concern.
4. It became increasingly evident that the trustees favored a sharp separation of the Health Plan and the Hospitals from the Medical Group.

"We are convinced to a man," they wrote further, that "separation would result in the destruction of everything we have achieved together. . . . We urge a return to these fundamental principles, not only for our own benefit, but for that of our successors and our imitators, and for what all of us believe to be an ideal of medical practice worth maintaining."[33]

Kaiser's response was pedestrian. He persisted in his letter-writing campaign and his usual patronizing tone with the doctors he considered in his employ. There was no meeting of the minds between Henry Kaiser and the Permanente physicians, for a reason clearly stated by several participants in the corporate-professional negotiations of 1955, among them George Link: "Mr. Kaiser was always thinking he was running [the medical program] . . . and [the doctors] thought they were running it. . . . One of the essential problems I think Mr. Kaiser as well as Gene Trefethen had, was a failure to recognize [the doctors'] professionalism . . . and their pride."[34]

The Working Council formed in May continued to meet for a few days each month, but none of the problems yielded to solution. The doctors persisted in their quest for autonomy and control of all medical affairs through operation and control of the health plan. Management saw that this was financially and legally impossible. Link gave his legal opinion to both sides. A reorganization would give the medical groups "control of the financial heart of the whole setup." Financial control would bring medical society charges against them of unethical solicitation of patients. Further, their control of health plan dues would jeopardize the tax-exempt status of the health plan and hospitals because the doctors would be operating for "personal financial gain" rather than "benefit of the community." Finally, loans for hospital construction continued to depend on the relationship between the Bank of America and Henry J. Kaiser, with Kaiser "morally responsible to pay the debt." Neither financiers nor Henry Kaiser would accept physician interference in financial affairs.[35]

While the doctors focused on professional philosophic issues, Kaiser and his deputies stuck to financial ones. They interspersed corporate opinions with a liberal dose of moralism. Though he did not attend Working Council meetings, Kaiser maintained personal involvement in the dispute. At times he patronized the physicians; at times he chastised them for financial greed. They had first asked for control of the health plan at the May council meeting. A week after the meeting and its flurry of demands and legal opinions, Kaiser drafted a dramatic "Dear Doctor" letter. He outlined the history of his program "to bring care to the people" as the greatest "goal of my life." Typically, he shifted from paternal good will to several imperious observations. The doctors would not be granted more control and direction of the Kaiser health plan and hospitals. This would endanger the financial structure, as well as abrogate the "public trust." The public trusted Kaiser not only because of his economic power, but also because the trustees had the strength to defend prepaid group practice "against the attacks of certain elements within organized medicine, competitive systems and even antagonistic political forces."[36] Kaiser refused to relinquish this impressive responsibility to the people.

Kaiser descended abruptly from grandiose idealism to penurious reality. If the medical groups insisted on operating the health plan and hospitals "in complete independence of us," then their activities would no longer be under Kaiser Foundation auspices. The trustees would sell all the facilities to the doctors and withdraw all legal and moral responsibility. If this is what the physicians wanted, they would have to make their own financial arrangements with the banks and pay off all indebtedness to the Kaiser Foundation "within a reasonable period of time such as six months."[37] He had suggested no less than an immediate severance of ties with the Northern California Permanente Medical Group.

Two weeks later Kaiser read another version of the letter to the rebellious doctors of the Working Council, giving them a lecture on competition. Separate, smaller partnerships would divide the rebelling physicians from those who were cooperative, breaking the power of medical group leaders. Kaiser no longer spoke of the groups collectively. It was clear, he said, that only "some members" of the groups demanded complete physician management of the hospitals and health plan. Those "segments" of the Permanente doctors who so desired this, Kaiser said dramatically, could arrange financing to purchase facilities that the doctors then would operate with total independence from the Kaiser Foundation and the "public trust." Referring to the May 12 memorandum from Baritell, Collen, Cutting, Kay, Neighbor, Saward, and Weiner three weeks before in which the doctors called the facilities "our Hospitals," Kaiser appeared shocked at their "error and mis-interpretations." "The several millions of dollars worth of Hospitals and facilities held in trust by the non-profit Founda-tion entities are NOT 'our hospitals'—neither yours, nor the Trustees'," he declared. "They belong to the public." Surely here he contradicted his own remarks at Walnut Creek in 1953, when he had clarified who in fact owned the hospital.[38]

The items numbered one to four in the memorandum, and the statement that "this organization was founded on the prin-ciples of integrated operations, under physician manage-ment," were of special concern to the industrialist. He continued to lecture on the meaning of a public trust. The medical groups were operated for private profit. Therefore, they could not manage and distribute funds from nonprofit, public trust facilities. The trustees would be guilty of malfea-sance and of conduct both morally and legally wrong if they surrendered their public trust to a profit-making entity. Kai-ser asserted that all the funds and assets were gifts from Kai-ser interests. They included funds of over $3 million derived from tax exemption and funds from bank loans granted only "because Henry Kaiser won't allow the bank to lose on the loans." It was impossible that these funds and assets could be "appropriated" by the dissidents for their own purposes. Therefore, those who desired physician management must ac-quire other facilities. Kaiser concluded his "statement" on a dramatic note: "I want to write all of the 500 or more doctors now serving Health Plan members . . . [that] we are not like old soldiers who just fade away; nevertheless we are prepared to step aside for the individual doctors who want us to bow out." They could create their own "private profit non-tax-exempt" plan, while Kaiser and the doctors who stayed could continue their medical work "in conjunction with the non-profit, public trust institutions."[39]

He "wanted them to know" many other things of a moral nature:

I do not concede that the Trustees would ever be a party to anything within our contract which—in your words—"would result in the destruction of everything we have achieved together." . . . I am sure you know that I will not participate in any dishonesty, any evasion, or any subterfuge. The ability of those of you who wish to go forward alone will free us to go forward with other work that is in our hearts to accomplish for the good of the people.[40]

Refusing financial support to the dissidents on the Working Council was the simplest and cleanest way for the trustees to divide the medical group leaders from the 500 other doctors they purported to represent.

The dissidents asked if they had to buy the facilities for cash or if "other reasonable methods of solving this particular problem may be considered." But Kaiser withdrew from the "discussion" as dramatically as he had entered it. Through Trefethen he informed the rebels that "within the spirit of his statement" they were free to work on any proposal but it "MUST LEAVE THE FOUNDATION FREE TO PROCEED WITH ITS OBJECTIVES." The next move was theirs; Kaiser had served notice that they must terminate their relationship to the medical care program if they could not work within the established structure. The "discussion" was ended.[41]

At one point in the exchange between Kaiser and the doctors, Morris Collen squared off with the powerful industrialist. Collen recalled the incident:

It was a small room. We were all around this table, and [Kaiser] leaned over and shook his fist right under my nose and said, "Collen, you want to take me on? Do you want to take me on?" My God, here I was a young physician and I didn't want to take him on! But we all had these firm principles that our [Permanente Medical Group] executive committee had agreed upon. We had to maintain our position of autonomy, and he didn't want that.[42]

The doctors did not want to leave the program. They moderated their tone, no longer mentioning control of the health plan. They switched to conciliatory statements, using "teamwork" in place of "integration" to define their goals. They also asked for increased financial and employment "security,"

which would "give incentive for doctors to provide high quality service." "Teamwork" committees were formed for each
region to meet at Kaiser's estate at Lake Tahoe on July 12,
1955.[43]

Kaiser left it up to Trefethen to work out an agreement.
Cutting characterized the difference in style of the two men
that made Trefethen the more likely to appease the physicians. Trefethen shared Kaiser's attitude that "anything we're
in, we run." He projected the image of a "hard manager,"
sometimes bombastic, pounding on the table during discussions. But unlike Kaiser he could be "calm" and was willing to
work on details. "Mr. Kaiser would come blustering in," Cutting said, "he was too busy to argue, you couldn't argue with
him. He would put his declaration down, and then get out. He
didn't want to be part of the nit-picking discussions . . . and
Mr. Trefethen had to sit there and take our abuse, and try to
present his conviction."[44]

Trefethen acknowledged the strength and passion of the
medical group representatives on the Working Council.
"Henry wants the doctors as employees, but that's not right,"
he said. "We really don't want the doctors as employees. We
want them as partners."[45] "These people get all emotionally
entangled with the subject, and you have to quiet them down,"
he said of Kay, Saward, and Collen. Trefethen "broke the ice"
with the simple idea of a contract between the two interest
groups. It would identify organizational roles, create an Advisory Council and Regional Management Teams so the program would be jointly administered, and change the structure
of revenue distribution, giving the doctors more "security"
and financial incentive. Over the next three years contracts
between the trustees and the medical groups were renegoti-
ated in each of the three regions.[46]

In June 1956 the Southern Permanente partners were first
to sign a contract with the Kaiser trustees. Trefethen credited
Raymond Kay's strong leadership and the fact that southern
California was experiencing most growth at the time for the
faster resolution in the south. "Kay was difficult" and sometimes "more emotional that the rest of them," Trefethen said.

But he was the dominant voice there. In northern California things would quickly "get out of hand" with leadership divided between Baritell, Collen, Cutting, and Garfield; "going down to Southern California I could talk to Ray Kay alone."[47]

Meanwhile local medical society antipathies dissolved. A cooperative investigation in 1954 by LACMA attorneys and Kay stilled the charge of lay interference in medical practice at Kaiser Permanente. Yet three more Los Angeles physicians were denied society membership in 1955, and Fontana physicians were turned down by the San Bernardino Medical Society. Kaiser lawyers advised against litigation. Legal actions would not stop the more subtle forms of discrimination that were the most damaging and would only escalate their use. Finally, in April 1956, Kay initiated a series of meetings with the LACMA attorney and Foster's successor, Dr. Ewing L. Turner. Turner told Kay that if he could "hold his guys back [from litigation] a couple of years," Turner "could get his board to come around. . . . We worked it out." Kay and Turner agreed that there was no legal or ethical justification for society rejection of Permanente doctors for membership, and they sought a compromise, short of a lawsuit, for their admission.[48] Turner's successors likewise were conciliatory. By the late 1950s Southern Permanente doctors were routinely accepted not only by the LACMA, the largest county society in the state, but by the smaller and more provincial San Bernardino society as well.

Problems with the societies in northern California were also resolved on an informal, personal level by Permanente and society leaders. The president of the San Francisco Medical Society, Dr. Samuel Sherman, advised in the society *Bulletin* that young doctors should not join closed-panel, prepaid medical groups. But there was no formal action against them if they did. When Collen became medical director at San Francisco in 1954, the Permanente group established a "liaison committee" with Dr. Bristol Nelson as chair; in Oakland, Dr. Robert King acted as the conciliator with the Alameda–Contra Costa County Medical Association. Both were distinguished obstetrician-gynecologists able to convince "the important people in the hierarchies of the local societies" to accept Permanente doctors. The societies never filed formal proposals or resolutions against Permanente.[49]

The Permanente doctors did not forget the sting of discrimination. Kay said that once medical association membership was routine, and though the Permanente group encouraged it, periodically offering to pay dues, "few of our physicians took advantage of the privilege" to join. Outside collegial acceptance meant more to some Permanente physicians than to others. Collen, for example, thought community involvement and prestige vital to his professional development in the medical research field. Other physicians such as Dr. Alice Friedman were uninterested.[50] Society membership was unnecessary. Permanente physicians did not rely on outside hospital privileges, nor did they need contacts in the collegial referral network to build their practices.

In mid-1957 Kay again had to rebut the editor of the LACMA regarding an article in the LACMA *Bulletin* critical of Southern Permanente. The author declared that most Kaiser health plan memberships were paid by employers and conferred unsolicited upon the individual patient as mandatory collective bargaining benefits preferred by union leaders and paternalistic management. These unwilling members tacitly rejected Kaiser care by continuing to see their own family doctors. The second indictment was that Kaiser owed its financial success to its nonprofit and therefore tax-exempt status. Private physicians enjoyed no such exemption. Finally, the *Bulletin* charged that despite the fact that Permanente doctors had a ready-made practice with captive patients provided by union leaders, had no overhead, had regular hours and other benefits of group practice, "there has been a tremendous turnover of disgruntled doctors."[51]

Kay countered with statistics. Although 40 percent of Kaiser Health Plan members did have their dues paid in whole or in part by employers, 60 percent were individual or group subscribers who paid for their own coverage, either directly or through salary deductions. No 100 percent groups had been accepted since the ILWU contract in 1950. "Dual choice" made it unnecessary for individuals to hold membership in

Kaiser when they had the choice of reimbursement through Blue Cross or other indemnity plans. The health plan was not tax exempt; only the Kaiser Foundation Hospitals had this status, like all other nonprofit voluntary hospitals, and for the same reasons, Kay continued. Finally, only 7 percent of Southern California Permanente physicians left for private practice between 1954 and 1957, not the vast numbers suggested by the *Bulletin*.[52]

Hints of tension with the societies in Oregon also were referenced in official records and papers. But Saward, like Kay, valued independence. He focused on the struggle with the Kaiser organization, including Garfield, rather than with the outside physician community in the region. Yet one Kaiser spokesperson later recalled that professional relations in Oregon were not even "reasonably satisfactory" until after 1961. Only after a "veiled threat" of antitrust litigation did the Multnomah County Medical Society begin to admit Permanente physicians. "Serious friction" in the less populated counties continued well into the 1970s.[53]

Saward did not wish to change the simple organizational structure set up in the Northwest region after the war. A single hospital and health plan corporation contracted with the Permanente Clinic for medical services; Saward continued to dominate both. His primary goal was a new hospital on the Portland side of the Columbia River. He finally obtained the promised construction of the Bess Kaiser Hospital in 1957, which Henry Kaiser exchanged for support of a health plan and hospital in Hawaii. The northern California group united behind Dr. Cecil Cutting, selected as executive director in 1957. In 1958 the group signed a contract with the trustees similar to the one adopted in southern California.[54]

Medical economist Michael Davis wrote in 1955 that the doctors' contract with the "nonprofit organization which is actually a by-product of the Kaiser industries" was "a useful device to mark the professional independence of the physicians."[55] Like the doctors' fight for acceptance by medical society colleagues, the medical service contracts between the Permanente groups and the Kaiser trustees had more symbolic than practical value. They based medical group income on the number of individual patients rather than on a percentage of membership dues—a token return to individualism in the doctor-patient relationship and a token of direct payment for care. The contracts also clearly separated the professional and corporate spheres of control within the organization through joint management in decentralized regional management teams led by the medical director, who acted also as the chief executive of the medical group. The regional manager was chief executive of hospital and health plan operations in each region.

The dual medical practice and lay management system clearly differentiated the professional from the nonprofessional medical program functions. Moreover, the contracts addressed the doctors' issues of economic security. The trustees promised program physicians a basic level of health plan revenue and split additional earnings on a fifty-fifty ratio. Along with other provisions for regional financial autonomy, the new contracts gave incentive for efficiencies and increased productivity on the local level. A retirement plan and other economic benefits recognized the practical bread-and-butter issues that made group practice attractive.[56] Most important, the contracts formally affirmed the doctors' professional autonomy and status.

Legal adviser George Link understood the significance of the contract for the doctors' professional pride and their desire "to run this thing on their own." Trefethen also acknowledged the contract as a symbolic declaration of equality. "What we finally agreed," he said, "was that we were 'partners,' that they had autonomy in medicine . . . and they would organize themselves, and run themselves, and we would contract with them on a per capita basis to handle the medical side of our health plan . . . and we would have a board of our own, and they would not be represented on it, and we would not be represented on their executive committees, or their boards." But Trefethen also adopted Kaiser's patronizing tone. The corporate interests were responsible, he said, for stimulating the doctors toward higher quality service by providing economic incentives.[57]

After the Lake Tahoe negotiations Henry Kaiser removed

Garfield and himself from active participation in the medical program on the West Coast, announcing that Garfield was "coming with me" to help with planning at Kaiser's new chosen community on Oahu, Hawaii. As he began the last decade of his life, Kaiser created a microcosm of the community that was elusive on the mainland. He built a small version of the integrated society he had begun on a grand scale during the depression and World War II. He fired Garfield, in a sense, and "took him away" to a new island frontier.[58] In 1955 Garfield was "relieved" of his administration of Kaiser Permanente. "All titles were stripped away," Clifford Keene recalled. For the next four years even Keene was placed on the payroll as "physician unclassified."[59]

Not for several years was the transition from Garfield's leadership to that of Keene given an official title. In 1957 and 1958, with expansion to Hawaii and construction of the Bess Kaiser Hospital in Portland, Keene described himself as "a general manager without title, job description or acknowledgement." Finally, in 1960, Keene was named a vice-president of Kaiser Industries, responsible for all Kaiser industrial-medical affairs and vice-president and general manager of the hospitals and health plan and their subsidiaries. "During the era of Mr. Henry Kaiser's central role," Keene observed, "there were very few titles . . . Henry was The Boss."[60]

The corporate-professional relationship was stabilized between 1956 and 1959 through decentralized leadership and the geographic withdrawal of Kaiser and Garfield. At the same time the AMA declared its truce with prepaid group practice in a special edition of the *JAMA* referred to as "the Larson Report." The AMA Committee on Medical Care for Industrial Workers officially approved labor clinics in 1954, but with major caveats. Clinic services could not compete with traditional practice by extending services beyond diagnosis or to higher paid workers and dependents.[61] The AMA could afford this magnanimity toward labor. In the middle 1950s union officials recognized the financial and logistic barriers for union medical clinics. It was unlikely that they would spread further. The overwhelming majority of union members with medical care benefits were enrolled in traditional insurance plans. In 1953 commercial carriers insured 29 percent of the U.S. population for hospital care, Blue Cross 27 percent, and independent plans only 7 percent.[62]

Statistics revealed the highly unusual medical situation that evolved in the San Francisco Bay Area due to Kaiser's presence, aggressive unionism, a "liberal political culture," and the volatile socioeconomic environment of the postwar period. While 70 percent of unionized workers were covered by negotiated health plans nationwide, 90 percent were covered in the Bay Area. Other aspects also differed markedly from the national pattern. A higher percentage of health care coverage was financed by collective bargaining (45 percent as opposed to 27 percent nationally). Also, only 62 percent of coverage was paid in full by employers nationally compared to 90 percent in the Bay Area.[63] The 141 local unions with members and dependents in the San Francisco Labor Council (AFL) represented one-half of the city's population, an enormous medical market.[64]

Kaiser refused to cooperate with other lay-sponsored health plans. After an initial enthusiasm in 1946 for the Health Insurance Plan of Greater New York, he declined participation with LaGuardia and other prominent HIP sponsors as well as other independent organizations combatting AMA restraint of trade. Kaiser agreed with Garfield's declaration in 1954 when asked to join a federation of group health plans fighting the AMA, that "we do not want to be identified with a militant organization fighting for the people's interests."[65]

Clifford Keene echoed this corporate conservatism. In reporting on HIP's annual meeting in 1956, Keene said he thought HIP was "wrong to fight the medical societies on 'free choice of physician.'" According to Keene, the "dual choice" approach, adopted by Kaiser officials as early as 1948, was the proven best response to the medical society charge that prepaid health plans denied free choice to their "captive patients."[66] The approach preserved the principles of voluntarism and competition, sacrosanct in the U.S. liberal economic tradition. Other prepaid group plans continued to fight Kaiser Permanente's battles against medical conservatives.

The long string of legal defeats combined with favorable

economic conditions, a physician shortage, and recognition by AMA leadership in the 1950s that lay-controlled prepayment plans were only a small threat nationally to prompt the profession to relax opposition to prepaid group health. Sociologist Paul Starr asserts that medical conservatives "gradually became reconciled to vigilant coexistence" with independent plans, including Kaiser.[67]

The Commission on Medical Care Plans, formed to study medical care plans in the wake of Resolution 16 at the AMA annual meeting in 1954, was chaired by Dr. Leonard W. Larson of Bismarck, North Dakota. Compromise was the commission's unspoken purpose, a dramatic reversal by the association from the previous decade. A veteran of such studies, Larson in 1950 chaired the AMA Medical Service Council's Correlating Committee on Relations with Lay-sponsored Voluntary Health Plans, when the most controversial issue on the agenda was whether these plans offered "free choice of physician."[68] Larson was from a midwestern rural state and expressed sympathy with the consumer cooperative movement, although he also recognized his obligation to uphold the professional philosophy and ethics of the AMA.

After that committee's work was completed in 1950, Larson discussed consumer-sponsored medical care plans "from the rural viewpoint." He was bitter about restrictions on freedom of speech and frustrated at the inability of the AMA to overcome the semantic barrier of "free choice of physician" whenever it considered the group plans. He chastised his colleagues for inflexibility. "Medicine is at the crossroads," he said, noting the incendiary political environment. "We are caught in the swirling tide of rapidly changing philosophies as to the responsibility of the state to the individual." He would agree with Henry Kaiser that such plans had the built-in safeguard of consumer choice. Adding a sprinkle of midwestern vernacular, he encouraged his colleagues "to take a squint down at the earth occasionally to see what is going on about us . . . no plan or scheme can succeed, even one based on compulsion, unless the consumer obtains the same high level of medical care which is so universally available in this country today."[69]

The Commission on Medical Care Plans placed voluntary

prepayment plans in three categories: medical society–approved plans, including Blue Shield; private indemnity insurance plans; and "miscellaneous and unclassified plans." The latter were set apart by their "method of payment to the physician" and their closed-panel nature. Only 6 percent of all persons with any type of insurance were covered by the 250 such plans that existed. The commission studied 107 of these, scrutinizing whether they were "lay-dominated" or controlled by physicians. Physician participation in policy decisions at the board and staff levels was the measuring stick for commission approval. Only 40 percent of the prepayment closed-panel plans met this requirement.[70] Permanente regional directors and group leaders affirmed this participation in the new medical service agreements negotiated with Kaiser simultaneously with the commission's study.

The commission found personnel and facilities provided by most of the plans "adequate," though spokespersons exaggerated the benefits of preventive medicine. But it criticized the weaknesses of the industrial medical programs among the unorthodox plans: their impersonality and dehumanization, and the corporate dominance over medical practice that invaded the most intimate recesses of workers' lives. The report blamed the big industrialist and labor union bosses such as Lewis and Bridges for their intrusion in the doctor-patient relationship. "Some unions," the report said, "believe that by organizing such plans they encourage a closer relationship between the member and the union." Management, too, saw the advantages of providing medical care benefits through collective bargaining: "a closer relationship between the employee and employer," "a more stabilized work force," and "reduced production loss." Physicians in prepaid group practice were totally absolved. Their patient care and professional dedication were judged equal with these qualities among independent fee-for-service practitioners. The report itemized the cases won against medical societies that had unjustly denied membership to physicians who participated in the prepayment group plans and warned the constituent societies of the grave consequences of disregarding the antitrust and libel laws.[71]

A decade after editor Morris Fishbein's resignation, the

JAMA report was an unmistakable gesture of reconciliation by the AMA toward colleagues in prepaid group practice. Moreover, the authors of the study admitted that low income groups did not enjoy "freedom of choice" in the private practice fee-for-service system. The unorthodox plans did "fill a definite need" among low income, unskilled, and semiskilled workers for basic health security.[72]

Permanente physicians and their traditionalist colleagues settled into an uneasy coexistence on the West Coast. Simultaneously, the personal management structure in California toppled, as Henry Kaiser retreated to Hawaii. A small management cadre of four or five men, led by Trefethen and comprised of medical economists and legal experts, was left as an embryonic "central office."[73]

In 1956 Henry Kaiser began moving his household and corporate headquarters permanently to the island of Oahu. He developed a new Kaiser community more tightly knit and geographically circumscribed than his farflung mainland medical-industrial empire. In semiretirement Kaiser turned increasingly to domestic and leisurely forms for expression of his entrepreneurial drive. He built a suburban community of modest middle-class homes at Hawaii Kai, a large resort hotel complex on Waikiki named "Hawaiian Village," and a health plan and medical center. Just as Kaiser and Garfield had begun their industrial communities in benign isolation in the desert West, Kaiser discovered a final frontier to develop at the westernmost extension of the nation. There he led one last battle against the AMA.

Creation of the Kaiser Permanente Hawaii Region in 1958, in opposition to the local medical community and strong advice of the mainland Permanente administrators, repeated a familiar scenario. In early 1955 the Hawaii Medical Association (HMA) appealed to Kaiser's "sense of fairness to not introduce a plan that has caused so much ill-will among doctors in the state communities where it has been located." Joined by the Honolulu County Medical Society, the HMA protested that there were enough hospital beds and that neither the doctors nor the people of Hawaii needed a Kaiser Health Plan on the islands. Kaiser responded with a personal lecture to the HMA House of Delegates to again educate traditional doctors in his "new medical economics," as well as to inform them of the needs and wishes of the Hawaiian people. He urged the society leaders to "initiate a freedom of choice" between their own fee-for-service indemnity plan (Hawaii Medical Service Association or HMSA) and the Kaiser prepaid group practice plan.

Kaiser said that thousands of Hawaiians had asked him to establish the plan in the islands. He designed a sixteen-story medical center in the spring of 1956 "as a consequence of the public requests."[74] He was under "almost constant pressure" by the AFL and ILWU to "inaugurate" his medical plan in Hawaii. The unions "almost demanded it." One floor would be devoted to multiphasic screening at a cost of only two to three dollars a year per member and to facilities for research in preventive medicine. Arthur A. Rutledge, president of the AFL Teamsters, and Hotel and Restaurant Workers, confirmed Kaiser's boast of union support. Just as the Alameda County society in northern California had done in the early 1940s, medical officials continued to protest that a hospital bed surplus existed and that Kaiser was neither needed nor wanted.[75]

Despite objections, Kaiser bulldozed ahead with his Hawaiian community building. At first he "expressly and intentionally" did not involve traditional leaders of the Permanente Medical Groups in his creation of a personal island health plan. In November 1956 Dr. Frederick Pellegrin, a veteran of the Walnut Creek conflict between Kaiser and the doctors, began househunting with his wife in Hawaii. Pellegrin was "working on a health plan format especially designed for Hawaii"; he initially expected 40,000 to 50,000 islanders to join. The Honolulu press reminded its readers that in January 1955 the HMA had "formally asked Mr. Kaiser not to introduce his health plan here, saying that it would 'create a great deal of dissension within the profession.'" Henry Kaiser suddenly fell silent about the project, apparently awaiting the eruption of the local doctors' furor. Never reluctant to go on the attack against the AMA, the ILWU characteristically took Kaiser's side. The union's English-language radio broadcast decried the AMA and local businesses for calling the Kaiser Medical Program "socialistic, of the creeping variety."[76]

Nine months later Kaiser held a press conference to announce the resumption of his medical facility plan, as lack of opposition in the press indicated to him that it now was acceptable to local doctors and viewed as a necessity by thousands of union members. HMA president Dr. Samuel L. Yee opposed him on the grounds that Kaiser Permanente did not abide by now-familiar ethical principles: "The free choice of physician and hospital by the patient should be preserved." Kaiser turned Yee's semantics back on him. He thought Yee's objection strange since HMSA was a "closed panel, open only to doctors who join it" and "all the doctors have not joined." "Am I wrong in my assumption?" Kaiser asked.[77]

The Kaiser Foundation Health Plan was established in Honolulu on May 21, 1958. The $4 million, 150-bed Kaiser Hospital was scheduled for completion at year's end. The *Hawaii Medical Journal* description of events dripped with sarcasm. The physician partnership formed to contract with Kaiser for medical services included some well-known local doctors: Yee, described as a general surgeon and past president of the HMA as well as of the Honolulu County medical and surgical societies; Dr. Homer M. Izumi, general practitioner, the HMA's former AMA delegate; Dr. W. B. Herter, pediatrician; Dr. Richard Durant, general surgeon and past president of the Honolulu County Medical Society; and Dr. Richard S. Dodge, orthopedic surgeon and first medical director of the Rehabilitation Center of Hawaii. Press reports stressed that the group would manage medical services "on a fully independent, autonomous basis" with mainland physicians brought in "only if the partnership so desires." It currently was open to all community physicians and all patients, whether or not they were plan members or insured by the HMSA. Group memberships would be available only on a "freedom of choice" basis.[78]

An "influential voice" in the "Island medical circle" expressed shock at the treason of the five local physicians, noting that three of the new partners had said they were not interested in Kaiser. He called for the resignations of Yee and Izumi from their HMA posts as AMA alternate delegate and councillor. The Honolulu County society president remarked: "I imagine anyone who changes his way of practice would do so for some kind of gain, like financial." Other doctors said they would refuse to practice at Kaiser even if their patients requested it.[79]

At first only Dr. Clifford Keene and legal executive Scott Fleming were involved in the "education" of Kaiser's Hawaiian doctors, who formed the Pacific Medical Associates (PMA) outside the Permanente Medical Group network. As a result of Henry Kaiser's daily personal involvement in its construction, the Honolulu Medical Center was completed between January and November 1958, and thirty-three additional staff physicians were employed by the PMA.[80]

The Hawaii Region had over 38,000 members within two years of operation, but in the spring of 1960, Kaiser's Hawaiian medical empire was in serious trouble. The PMA physicians concentrated on their independent practices rather than on developing the new Kaiser program. According to Scott Fleming, "None of them really understood group practice, and the operation was functioning more as a collection of physicians in one location than as an organized medical group." Moreover, they demanded major increases in financial reimbursement, placing all financial responsibility on Kaiser as a bottomless funding source. While service complaints and discrimination in favor of private patients escalated in mid-1960, the partners issued an "ultimatum" to Kaiser to increase their compensation, "or else."[81]

In August 1960 Henry Kaiser told the press that the five doctors had repudiated and terminated their contract after "more than nine months of fruitless efforts to persuade them to live up to their obligations." They had "enriched themselves" and refused to carry out program principles at the expense both of plan members and of other group physicians. They had made "astoundingly excessive demands" that were "utterly and fantastically ridiculous and impossible." They received personal net incomes of $50,000 a year each, the equivalent, Kaiser said, of $100,000, since solo practitioners spent up to 50 percent of patient fees in office space, equipment, and personnel. Kaiser accused PMA Medical Director Dodge of saying, "If Mr. Kaiser has to borrow another half million dollars [to pay the doctors], let him do it and pay us what we want." What they wanted was an increase to $60,000 a year in individual salaries. Pounding on the table, Dr. Durant had told health plan officials, "By God, this is our final offer and you will meet it or else!" On August 19, 1960 the partners were informed that their "or else" ultimatum constituted repudiation of their health plan contract, and they must vacate the premises in twenty-four hours.[82]

A powerful team of Kaiser medical and lay executives that included Keene, Saward, Fleming, and medical economist Arthur Weissman arrived on the scene to bail out their floundering elder chieftain. With the firm hand that Henry Kaiser had lost, they gave the recalcitrant doctors written notice to vacate the premises within a day's time. The remaining thirty-three doctors were reorganized under the leadership of Dr. Philip Chu and Saward's mentorship as the Hawaii Permanente Medical Group. Saward remained executive consultant. The mainland Kaiser Permanente team finally brought order to Henry Kaiser's last medical care frontier.[83]

The influence and direction of Kaiser and Garfield waned in the middle 1950s as the new group of legal advisers, medical economists, regional managers, and business-oriented medical leaders turned the program onto its contemporary course. Yet the two program founders could rest on their laurels in Henry Kaiser's new island community, where their mutual affection increased. Though there is little of Garfield's own written record of this unique relationship, a brief note from Henry Kaiser to his "personal physician" indicates its depth. In response to Garfield's lament that he no longer "controlled" the vast medical empire they had created, Kaiser gently reminded him of his still active role, especially in facilities design. "Too bad, Sid," wrote the aging industrialist, "you have nothing to do and don't control anything! It looks to me like I'll have to find something else for you to do as these duties apparently are not enough. I'll have you fix my foot in the morning." The note ended, "All my love, Henry J. Kaiser."[84]

Though Kaiser was persuaded by Eugene Trefethen and

Edgar Kaiser to replace Garfield with Clifford Keene, and though he recognized the need for the shift of authority, Kaiser never accepted Keene on a personal level. For the remaining decade of his life, Kaiser complained to Trefethen and Edgar of Keene's imperious and undiplomatic attitude and his intrusions into Kaiser's own Hawaii Region. Kaiser's belief that the Hawaii Region would be his personal medical community despite its obvious faltering in regard to membership growth and the development of a strong physicians' group made him resist the involvement of the new cadre of physician executives in his island retreat.

While Keene, Saward, and others worked to straighten out problems in Hawaii, Kaiser expressed his displeasure to Trefethen. Once he wrote, "To find Dr. Keene is over here without any discussion with me with reference to it, I feel very distressed." Completely discounting the radical overthrow of Kaiser's own physician group, and the necessity to reform the medical group and set the program on an upward course in membership and financial stability, Kaiser continued:

Dr. Keene had this responsibility [of improving Honolulu Health Plan membership] for nearly a year and did not accomplish anything. You know, Gene, I am fearful of the damage that Dr. Keene can do by the use of his poor judgment. We've had several unquestionable evidences in this in the past year . . . I feel badly to think that I was as responsible as anyone for bringing Dr. Keene into the picture, and because of my mistake in this regard, I do not want failures of the past repeated.

Apparently Kaiser knew he was on shaky practical ground in his criticism of Keene. Trefethen was the only one whom the usually vociferous and demanding Kaiser informed of his displeasure. He somewhat childishly proclaimed he would take up Keene's conduct neither with the Hawaii Regional Manager nor with Dr. Keene, "since [Keene] had failed."[85]

Beginning in late 1953 Clifford Keene had the thankless task of carrying forward the Kaiser Foundation Hospitals and Health Plan as they had evolved since the late 1930s. Keene's dedication remained firm despite the difficulty of his role as a lightning rod for years of acrimony between the opposing corporate and professional interests. Keene accepted his position in the "bad graces of Mr. Kaiser," believing that the contribution Kaiser had asked him to make to the program as a whole was more important than Kaiser's personal dislike. "In spite of the tumult and the shouting," Keene later wrote, "I did do the job that [Kaiser] brought me west to do and I did it exactly as he himself told me how he wanted it done on that night at Edgar's house in November 1953." Concerned to set the historic record straight, Keene also pointed out that "Mr. Kaiser's relationship with anyone I knew always went through a honeymoon, brief marriage, and then intense disillusionment."[87] Yet Keene recognized his own significance in the history of U.S. health care during the second half of the twentieth century:

Without and with various titles I was the fiscal manager of Kaiser Permanente from 1958 to 1975. At the time of his death in 1967, Mr. Kaiser's medical creation was the most successful enterprise of its kind in the world. Moreover it had achieved tranquility within itself and with the world at large. I thank Mr. Kaiser for giving me the opportunity to do large things in American medicine.[86]

Sidney Garfield escaped Kaiser's wrath at the end. Keene did not. He was less reluctant than the unquestioning Garfield to articulate his impressions of Kaiser, who appeared to retreat in his final years into a garrulous patriarch presiding over his self-contained, geographically isolated island oasis.

From the late 1950s until his death in 1967 at age eighty-five, Henry Kaiser was the grain of sand in the oyster—an irritant that produced a unique creation. Kaiser Permanente survived and prospered after its first two decades, a blueprint for the proliferation of the prepaid group practice plans that permanently altered the shape of medicine in the United States.

Conclusion

IN ITS FIRST TWO DECADES, Kaiser Permanente development reflected the dual paradox of corporate-professional conflict and social unrest woven throughout this study. First, one of the most expansive capitalists in the mid-twentieth-century United States created a private corporate welfare system supported by the political Left in the union movement and among public health and consumer activists. Liberal Democrats of the Roosevelt and Truman administrations also advocated the Kaiser plan. These groups were to the left of the Kaiser boardroom, however, and sought more far-reaching reform through government action. They brought their reform agenda to fruition in the Medicare and Medicaid legislation of the mid-1960s, under the Democratic Lyndon B. Johnson (LBJ) administration.

The health legislation of LBJ's Great Society precipitated an economic crisis in medical care beyond the conservatives' worst fears. Catastrophic inflation of costs was fueled rather than alleviated by the combination of Medicare and Medicaid and traditional insurance. From 1950 to 1965 per capita health care expenditures increased less than 8 percent a year. They rose to over a 14 percent annual increase after 1965. Between 1965 and 1970, government expenditures on the state and federal levels rose 20.8 percent yearly, increasing from $10.8 billion to $27.8 billion.[1] Conservative Republicans, returned to power with the Nixon administration, coopted liberals in the prepaid group health movement to develop an antidote to the crisis. Administration policy analysts reframed the concepts of prepaid group health in the HMO Act of 1973. Henry Kaiser's brand of welfare capitalism—rather than the prepaid plans envisioned by consumer cooperatives, welfare labor unionists, and liberal physicians—was the prototype for the new legislation, which had a history dating to World War II.

The period 1943 through 1946 was a turning point in the redefinition of social and economic relations in U.S. medicine. Two powerful messages emerged from the litigation that proceeded for a decade after the 1943 Group Health Association triumph in court over the AMA for "restraint of trade." The ruling symbolized the waning of physicians' cultural authority in U.S. society and presaged a complete realignment of social and economic relations in the country's medicine. It redefined the terms of the debate between the unorthodox health plans and the medical societies, opening the field to innovation and legitimizing a liberal economic language of health reform. Supported both by welfare capitalists and unionists, the U.S. justice system permanently damaged the AMA's public image. It shifted the arena of combat for reform from incendiary ideological symbols to the bread-and-butter terms of economic behavior.

Medicine was defined as a business that served consumers, subject to the same free enterprise regulations as other areas of commerce and industry. The language of the marketplace expressed a new doctor-patient contract that replaced paternalism and dependency based on "trust" with contractual equality and mutual responsibility in the healing process. Medicine was demystified, the facade of the physician stripped to a more human face.[2] Images of the doctor in the popular press also diminished the physician's image. At best they were small-town shop proprietors; at worst they were capitalists operating on principles of economic individualism contrary to the public interest.[3]

Finally, the 1959 Federal Employees' Health Benefits (FEHB) Act affirmed Kaiser Permanente's competitive principles and acceptance of private sector reform as a substitute for the centralized public welfare state adopted by other industrial nations. The influx of half a million federal government and state workers to Kaiser after the passage of the act and the California state employees benefit program rose steadily.[4]

Despite the ideological radicalism of some Permanente physicians and unionists like Harry Bridges, neither Henry Kaiser nor Sidney Garfield was left of center in the political arena. Neither sought significant social change. Their incremental, pragmatic goals contrasted with the aims of those who sought broader reform. The Kaiser trustees spoke the same language as mainstream physicians who opposed socialized medicine. Privatized prepaid group practice was a much lesser evil than state- or union-controlled medicine. Corporate political centrism was a bridge to truce with medical conservatives.

Opposed by virtually all other interest groups in U.S. politics, the AMA declared reluctant peer acceptance of their colleagues in prepaid group practice in the Larson Report. Local medical society antagonism also withered gradually. The regional economy contributed to the uneasy truce between Kaiser Permanente and its county medical society opponents by the late 1950s. It appeared that the Kaiser economic threat receded. A contemporary Berkeley labor economist may have comforted local doctors by asserting that Kaiser's growth pattern was "extensive" rather than "intensive," occurring through expansion into new geographical territory rather than monopoly in the areas where it operated. By 1959 the communities of largest Kaiser expansion had little more than one-fifth of the total population enrolled. The analyst predicted that, in California, the rapid increase of an upwardly mobile population created enough demand for private care on the traditional model to fill both the Kaiser Foundation Health Plan rolls and the offices of private practitioners.[5]

By 1953 Kaiser economists estimated that eighty-five million people had some degree of medical insurance coverage. About thirty-eight million were enrolled in Blue Cross, twenty-four million in commercial group insurance plans, and eighteen million through individual insurance policies. Only five million were covered by "other types of plans" that usually combined prepayment and group practice.[6] True competition by the prepaid group practice plans with the Blue Cross–Blue

Shield and the commercial insurance network was a factor only in a few areas, such as the Kaiser Permanente Pacific state regions. Yet the Kaiser Permanente plan remained a powerful local threat to independent doctors. The sanguine predictions of the late 1950s were overly optimistic for solo fee-for-service practitioners in Kaiser regions, especially in northern California. Indemnity insurance and fee-for-service practice were geared to the middle class, practical only for those with incomes over $2500 a year and workers with group policies subsidized by employers.[7] Even though these traditional forms continued to prevail, the medical market in northern California moved persistently toward Kaiser.

Kaiser Permanente attracted growing public support because it filled a critical gap in the welfare infrastructure. Government, the medical profession, and the insurance industry failed to reduce medical cost barriers for working-class and middle income families. At the same time these families made more demands on the health system because of ever-rising expectations of medical "progress" and biotechnology. In 1958 total Kaiser membership was 618,000; in 1959, 690,000; and in 1960, 808,000.[8] The anticorporate competitive strategy of the local medical establishment, first launched with the California Physicians' Service in 1939, failed to slow Kaiser expansion. The *San Francisco Chronicle* declared Kaiser Permanente the winner "hands down" of the "marketing battle for Northern California health care dollars in the 1980s."[9]

By 1990 the Kaiser Foundation Health Plan provided coverage for one-third of the population of San Francisco, as well as of Santa Rosa and Vallejo; for 37 percent of Oakland, the largest regional penetration nationally; 24 percent of Sacramento; 21 percent of Hawaii; 26 percent of Vancouver, Washington; and 19 percent of Portland, Oregon. Growth in southern California leveled out after the rapid growth at mid-century. In 1990 14 percent of the population of the Los Angeles, Long Beach, and Ventura area belonged to the health plan after four decades. Kaiser membership remained similar to that of the post–World War II period. Of 1990 members, 58 percent were from private sector employer groups; the next largest proportion was government employees, with 18 percent from state and local government, and 9 percent from the federal bureaucracy; 5 percent were in education, and only 10 percent were individuals not affiliated with a large group enrollment.[10]

In many ways Kaiser Permanente was a typical compromise among competing interests in twentieth-century U.S. society to produce a hybrid creation. In addition to providing a case study of Paul Starr's analysis of the "transformation" from individualized to corporate organization, Kaiser Permanente cut across traditional socioeconomic relations, inverting the institutional structures described in recent studies.[11] Its goals of access and economy in community care, rather than inwardly directed biomedical research and technological development, reversed the familiar social and institutional ranking in the U.S. medical system.

Accordingly, the Permanente physician profile differed markedly from tradition. In the the early 1930s, as Garfield started his contract medical practice on the southern California desert, county physicians suffered intense status anxieties in their local practice environments, as the traditional community welfare structures collapsed in the Great Depression.[12] At the same time, the early Permanente physicians were excluded by their colleagues in the AMA county societies and by elite medical academics. These factors caused psychological and social pressures in the profession, exacerbated by Henry Kaiser's meddlesome and autocratic behavior toward doctors inside and outside his medical program. But Permanente physicians faced events much larger than Kaiser's trouble making. They were the first to experience the upheaval in their profession, in the transition from solo fee-for-service practice to large prepaid group plans that grew rapidly in the last quarter of the century.

The deference and paternalism in traditional medicine first fully clashed with the egalitarianism of the labor and consumer movements at midcentury. Kaiser effected a practical resolution. Kaiser organizers operated on strict business principles while seeking to maintain traditional values of community. However, Kaiser eliminated charity from the community values of health care institutions, while adding concepts of a mutual participatory community of care for working-class and middle income patients. In the Kaiser Permanente system the doctor-patient relationship rests on equal responsibility for maintaining health. This mutual responsibility replaces the "gift relation" characteristic of traditional patriarchal European welfare systems.[13]

Ironically, however, Permanente doctors had to endure the patriarchal arrogance of Henry Kaiser at the same time that they abdicated their personal authority over patients. Not until the literal withdrawal of the forceful Kaiser and the creative Garfield from day-to-day program management did the dust settle over the turbulent organizational environment. A new cadre of modern managers neutralized interpersonal conflict and the clash of powerful personalities.

The pragmatic Henry Kaiser had shown more respect for the independence of the working-class family than for the professional autonomy of the Permanente physicians, a consequence of his own cultural identity. He was a populist, a man of little education and no elitist pretense. In Kaiser's mind the physicians were employees. Industrial workers had the more elevated status as producers and consumers of material goods and services, including the commodity of medical care. Moreover, the mechanistic language of "health maintenance" did not hold derogatory connotations for technologically inclined Americans at midcentury. They were not offended by references to their bodies as well-oiled machines. Patients accepted the goal of quality maintenance in order to gain full benefit from the natural life of their organic systems.[14] In the Kaiser boardroom mass production was the organizational priority.

The medical groups were led by physicians from a pragmatic rather than theoretical base in social medicine. Garfield had himself come from a midwestern academic institution at which the discipline of sociology was translated to a "meliorist" service program adjusted to contemporary local needs. At the University of Southern California, with which he later affiliated, sociology was conceived as "a social work program with strong practical emphases" rather than as a theoretical intellectual discipline. Other Permanente leaders likewise received their education in the new centers of social science of the

1920s. Morris Collen attended the University of Minnesota; Cutting was a graduate of Stanford. Later Saward left Northern Permanente to be a professor of social medicine at the University of Rochester, the institution at which he earned his medical degree. A second wave of public health ideologues brought turmoil in the early 1950s, represented by Weinerman of Yale.[15]

Large numbers of unorthodox physicians adopted Permanente social priorities in medicine. Despite the embarrassment some suffered from Henry Kaiser's public posturing and from rejection by their independent colleagues, increasing numbers of physicians joined the Permanente group partnerships. By 1955 only about 5 percent of all U.S. physicians, less than an estimated 10,000 of the 218,061 physicians, were engaged in group practice. Five hundred of them joined the Permanente Medical Groups, serving 523,510 members of the Kaiser Foundation Health Plan on the West Coast.[16]

By the time of Henry Kaiser's death in 1967 Kaiser Permanente was heralded by government and top medical analysts as the largest, most popular, and most financially successful prepaid group practice plan in the nation, sharing the spotlight in scale only with the Health Insurance Plan of Greater New York. HIP had a comparably large membership but lacked Kaiser's structural integration. Its doctors were spread among twenty to thirty groups, who used outside hospitals. In 1955 Kaiser had an estimated 50,000 more members than HIP; it was 3.5 times larger than Ross-Loos and almost 24 times larger than the Group Health Association. Of 150 prepaid group practice plans covering about four million people in the early 1960s, Kaiser Permanente and HIP had almost half of the total subscribers.[17]

The key regional leaders were idealistic in their view that the advantages in efficiency and the ability to treat more patients for less money served social welfare goals not met by the independent solo practice system. Permanente doctors received their own benefits as well: regular hours, more family time, and financial security. Permanente accepted only about one of every eight recruits in the early 1950s. Membership continued to grow 10 percent annually in California into the early 1960s, after a decade of twentyfold growth from 1945 through the middle 1950s; a new Permanente doctor joined the medical groups for each 1,000 new members. Yet the physician turnover rate from termination, retirement, and death remained at only about 7 percent a year.[18]

A 1967 federal government study indicated that a professional self-monitoring system had developed from the unique Permanente medical culture that replaced the fee-for-service and individual patient choice traditionally relied upon by physicians for professional control of quality and ethics. It was a process built into group practice in which doctors routinely reviewed the work of colleagues to maintain a high caliber of performance among the medical group physicians.[19]

The federal study noted a low rate of hospitalization as the primary program efficiency. This resulted from a cautious, cost-conscious assessment of individual patient needs within the framework of a strong outpatient care program. The ILWU multiphasic screening begun in 1951 for large member groups represented the juxtaposition of the liberal social welfare philosophy with innovative clinical methods that made the program successful with large working-class groups. It demonstrated commitment to public health concepts of community education, information, and a social medicine philosophy of preventive, comprehensive care for working Americans and their families. The emphasis at Kaiser on outpatient treatment rejected reliance on orthodox hospital practice.

Nationally, outpatient visits increased fourfold between 1956 and the early 1980s, while inpatient hospitalization increased only 2.5 times. Yet analysts still cited excessive hospitalization as the major factor contributing to the financial crisis in health care. In the late twentieth century hospitalization still meant a traditional medical practice environment. Insurance companies continued to reimburse doctors and hospitals more readily for inpatient than for outpatient treatment. Studies three decades after the ILWU multiphasic project showed that traditional hospital staff and physicians had no persuasive incentive to prevent hospital stays or to reduce their length. The result was that an estimated 20 percent of hospitalizations was "unnecessary."[20]

The emphasis on ambulatory care and large reduction in hospitalization for diagnosis and treatment, as well as frugality in administrative costs, were the two major economies emphasized by Kaiser Permanente. Like other social benefactors, the Kaiser family followed the traditional philanthropies in their focus on material monuments to their largess. But this attitude did not lead to nearly the traditional degree of institutional confinement. A 1957–58 health care survey under the Steelworkers' contract found that the union families who were members of Kaiser Permanente, HIP, GHA, and Group Health Cooperative of Puget Sound had only 60 percent of the number of hospital days as those enrolled in Blue Cross.[21] Per capita medical care costs, adjusted for age, rose over 19 percent in the California Kaiser Foundation Health Plan, from 1960 to 1965, but 43.5 percent in the nation as a whole. Again the difference was attributed to conservative hospitalization at Kaiser.[22]

Unlike hospitals in older regions of the nation, Kaiser hospitals have followed the massive decentralization of its membership in the 1950s away from central cities. Kaiser regions function autonomously yet within a unified framework, each planned to mirror regional demographics. Unlike the fragmented independent hospital system, Kaiser combined the virtues of local autonomy with those of national planning.

After 1959 and the large influx of government workers, Kaiser Permanente entered a third phase of development, an era of rapid yet stable expansion.[23] When Henry Kaiser died in 1967, Kaiser Permanente had twenty-nine clinics and fifteen hospitals in the Northern California, Southern California, Oregon, and Hawaii regions, serving about 1.5 million members. The program grew to cover a portion of the population for most of the island of Oahu, Hawaii, in 1969, and was extended to Maui within two years of Kaiser's death. Also in 1969 Kaiser Permanente began an aggressive expansion program eastward, with formation of the Ohio and Colorado regions.

In the last decade of the twentieth century, the program covered new regions in all sections of the United States: Texas, Kansas and Missouri, Georgia, North Carolina, Connecticut, Massachusetts, New York, and the Washington, D.C., and Baltimore areas. Within twenty years of Henry Kaiser's death, unforeseen even by the empire builder, the Kaiser Permanente program was indeed a national model for the large number of health maintenance organizations that sprang up in the 1970s and 1980s. While the national HMO census dropped from 650 separate health maintenance plans in 1988 to 575 in 1990, in the Northern California Region the Kaiser Foundation Health Plan increased to more than 2.4 million members, one-third of the regional population. The next largest HMO had only 134,000. Even with unprecedented rate increases over the next two years of 19.6 and 18 percent, Kaiser Permanente rates remained an average of 12 percent lower than those of other HMOs, and 20 to 30 percent lower than those of traditional indemnity insurance.[24]

In its early development Kaiser Permanente leaders parodied the traditional U.S. system of "community hospitals" and solo practitioners. To counter opposition its leaders adopted traditional semantics of "free choice," personal doctor-patient relations, and emphasis on the suburban family. But the program substituted important elements of scale, financing, and purpose that diverged from the "charitable" purpose of the independent "voluntary" hospital supported by Hill-Burton in 1946, and by the Medicare and Medicaid legislation of 1965. Its medical centers were much larger than the national average in number of beds, on the large scale of public hospitals (see table 5.1). Their size was a response to burgeoning membership and to emphasis on humanistic medical economics and efficiencies rather than the mass institutionalization of the dependent poor characteristic of public policy. The health plan sought to dignify rather than degrade patients who paid their own way.

The official definition of HMOs was both contradictory and ambiguous. At the end of 1973, the year of passage of the HMO Act, a *Health/Pac Bulletin* described them as health care organizations "intended to provide comprehensive services to a voluntarily enrolled membership at a prepaid fixed price." The definition left out the vital facilities and full-time group practice Garfield insisted were integral to success. There were further critical deviations from the Kaiser Permanente model. An HMO could be "funded privately, publicly or be a combination of both; it may be for-profit or non-profit." Doctors could practice full-time or part-time with the HMO and could be salaried or paid fee-for-service. By the end of 1973 there were over sixty so-called HMOs with eight million subscribers in a patchwork combination of prepaid group and fee-for-service rate systems, some with their own hospitals, some centered only around Independent Practice Associations.[25]

These definitions of the HMO bore little resemblance to the pragmatic operating principles developed by early Kaiser Permanente organizers, or to the social medicine philosophy of the ideologues among Permanente physicians.[26] In the Kaiser Permanente lexicon, doctor-patient equality was integral to the economic imperative for consumer satisfaction on the free market. Competition for the business of the patient consumer, or the member of a freely chosen health plan, placed the patient in the active role essential to successful practice of preventive medicine. Garfield, Kaiser, and their associates rejected tradition, and they adapted the language of public health, social, and preventive medicine to the practical demands of U.S. society in the second half of the twentieth century.

Notes

Introduction

1. Myrl Nygren and Alred W. Childs, *Kaiser and the Federal Employees' Health Benefits Program* (Berkeley: University of California Institute of Business and Economic Research, 1974), vii. The Kaiser family adopted the title "Permanente" from the old Spanish name for a creek near the company's Santa Clara cement plant south of San Francisco Bay. Mark S. Foster, *Henry J. Kaiser: Builder in the Modern American West* (Austin: University Texas Press, 1989), pp. 65–66; Sidney R. Garfield interview by Foster, January 16, 1984. Garfield died in February 1985.

2. The act gave planning grants and other benefits to federally qualified HMOs and superseded all state law restricting corporate medicine.

3. Kaiser Permanente, *Annual Report 1988–1989* (Oakland, Calif., 1989) and *Facts 1990* (Oakland, Calif., 1990). Sabin Russell, "Kaiser's Rates to Climb 19%," San Francisco *Chronicle*, Business Extra, 25 September 1989, C1; Russell, "Kaiser Rate Rises Amid HMO Turmoil," *ibid.*, 27 August 1990, C1.

4. Winslow quoted in Arthur J. Viseltear, "Compulsory Health Insurance and the Definition of Public Health," in Ronald L. Numbers, ed., *Compulsory Health Insurance—The Continuing Debate* (Westport, Conn.: Greenwood, 1982), 27. From C.-E. A. Winslow, "The Untilled Fields of Public Health," *Modern Medicine* 2:1 (1920).

5. Sidney R. Garfield, "The Kaiser Co. Makes It Work," *Fortune*, January 1945, 18.

6. Scott Fleming interview by author, 16 March 1989, Oakland, Calif.

7. Michael Kazin, "The Great Exception Revisited: Organized Labor and Politics in San Francisco and Los Angeles, 1870–1940," *Pacific Historical Review* 55 (1986), 371–402; Gerald D. Nash, *The American West Transformed: The Impact of the Second World War* (Bloomington: Indiana University Press, 1985), 5, 9, 19.

8. Joan B. Trauner, "From Benevolence to Negotiation: Prepaid Health Care in San Francisco, 1850–1950" (Ph.D. diss., University of California, San Francisco, 1977), 1–5; William Issel, "Liberalism and Urban Policy in San Francisco from the 1930s to the 1960s," *Western Historical Quarterly* 22:4 (November 1991), 431–450.

9. Alan Derickson, *Workers' Health, Workers' Democracy: The Western Miners' Struggle, 1891–1925* (Ithaca, N.Y.: Cornell University Press, 1988), x–xii; from AMA, Council on Medical Education and Hospitals, "Hospital Service in the United States," *JAMA* 76 (1921), 1083; Trauner, "From Benevolence to Negotiation," 6–7; cf. J.B. de C. M. Saunders, "Geography and Geopolitics in California Medicine," *Bulletin of the History of Medicine* 41 (1967), 293–324. Trauner refers to a California Medical Association survey, "Physician Supply in California, December 1973," in *Socioeconomic Report* 15:1–6 (1975). It indicates that the same demographics continued to the year of passage of the HMO Act. Los Angeles County had the largest number of active, nonfederal physicians in the state, 14,346, or 206.7 per 100,000 residents. San Francisco County, with 3,587 physicians, had the highest concentration, 530.9 per 100,000 residents. For the state as a whole the ratio was only 185.9 to 100,000.

10. See Edward D. Berkowitz and Wendy Wolff, *Group Health Association: A Portrait of a Health Maintenance Organization* (Philadelphia: Temple University Press, 1988), 3–15, for shifting occupational class roles within GHA. Daniel M. Fox places biomedical research, biotechnology, and medical education at premier institutions at the apex of regional medical systems in *Health Policies, Health Politics: The British and American Experience, 1911–1965* (Princeton, N.J.: Princeton University Press, 1986), ix–xi.

11. In 1940 only 2,093 physicians were engaged in full-time group practice; in 1950, about 5,000, but only 2.6% of U.S. doctors; by 1959, 5.2%. In a 1988 AMA survey almost 47% responding physicians practiced in groups of two or more; but 60% of AMA physicians reported a substantial part of their income from the Preferred Provider Organizations, Independent Practice Associations, and other "managed care" arrangements from which most U.S. workers and their families obtained medical service. Employers reported 96% of insured workers enrolled in traditional fee-for-service and indemnity health plans in 1984; in 1988, 28%. AMA Center for Health Policy Research, *Physician Marketplace Statistics 1989*, 85 (table 52); "Can You Afford To Get Sick?" *Newsweek*, September 30, 1989, 47. Estimate of physicians engaged in managed care from a special study by the Council on Long Range Planning and Development, *JAMA*, 1987.

12. Garfield numbered 300 prepayment plans in 1944 in "Health Plan Principles in the Kaiser Industries," *JAMA* 126 (7 October 1944), 338–339. The AMA identified nearly 250 in 1955, with the largest numbers in New York and California. See AMA, Commission on Medical Care Plans, "Special Report," part 2, appendix C, *JAMA* (17 January 1959). For early American hospitals: Charles E. Rosenberg, *The Care of Strangers: The Rise of America's Hospital System* (New York: Basic Books, 1987); David Rosner, *A Once Charitable Enterprise: Hospitals and Health Care in Brooklyn and New York, 1885–1915* (Princeton, N.J.: Princeton University Press, 1982); Morris J. Vogel, *The Invention of the Modern Hospital: Boston, 1870–1930* (Chicago: University of Chicago Press, 1980). For European health systems: Deborah A. Stone, *The Limits of Professional Power: National Health Care in the Federal Republic of Germany* (Chicago: University of Chicago Press, 1980), 20–27. The German Bismarckian system was, Stone states, "to solidify worker loyalty to the state." All blue-collar workers and those under a certain income level were required to belong to a "sickness fund." The state shared control of the funds with over 1,400 workers' associations descended from medieval artisan guilds. "National efficiency" was the rationale for the British system.

The formal discipline of social medicine incorporated eugenics concepts in the 1930s and 1940s, and the desire for class control through the welfare state. See Dorothy Porter and Roy Porter, "What Was Social Medicine? An Historiographical Essay," *Journal of Historical Sociology* 1:1 (April 1988), 90–106. Also, Charles Webster, *The Health Services Since the War*, vol. 1: *Problems of Health Care—The National Health Service Before 1957* (London: Her Majesty's Stationery Office, 1988).

13.   Rosenberg, *The Care of Strangers*, 33–34, 36; Trauner, "From Benevolence to Negotiation," 22–26; George Rosen, *Preventive Medicine in the United States, 1900–1975* (New York: Science History Publications, 1975), 20–29. From 1798 to 1870 all merchant seamen had a monthly payroll deduction of twenty cents; from 1870 to 1884, forty cents. Congress repealed the hospital tax on seamen in 1886, shifting it to a shipowners' tax based on tonnage. In 1905 Congress authorized direct appropriations for the service.

14.   Trauner, "From Benevolence to Negotiation," 4–7.

15.   Jerome L. Schwartz, "Early History of Prepaid Medical Care Plans," *Bulletin of the History of Medicine* 39 (September–October 1965), 456; Trauner, "From Benevolence to Negotiation," 2–3, 17–19.

16.   Western labor health historians are Trauner, "From Benevolence to Negotiation," 4–7, 19–30; Derickson, *Workers' Health, Workers' Democracy*, x–xiii; Schwartz, "Early History of Prepaid Plans," 450–475, on the prevalence of contract practice in Washington and Oregon. Rosemary Stevens, *In Sickness and In Wealth: American Hospitals in the Twentieth Century* (New York: Basic Books, 1989), 173, for large percentage of hospital deaths in the West.

17.   Rickey Hendricks, "History of UCSF," unpublished paper, 1990; Trauner, "From Benevolence to Negotiation," 6–7; Saunders, "Geography and Geopolitics," 293–324; Derickson, *Workers' Health, Workers' Democracy*, x–xiii; Paul Starr, *The Social Transformation of American Medicine* (New York: Basic Books, 1982), 170, for proprietary hospitals.

18.   Trauner, "From Benevolence to Negotiation," 163; Arnold I. Kisch and Arthur J. Viseltear, *The Ross-Loos Medical Group* (U.S. Public Health Service: Washington, D.C., 1967); Berkowitz and Wolff, *Group Health Association*, 47–54, 178.

19.   Special Report, *JAMA*, part 1(17 January 1959), 6.

20.   "U.S. Medicine in Transition," *Fortune*, December 1944, 157. An AMA survey revealed that 63% of doctors in uniform preferred a form of practice other than traditional solo fee-for-service practice; 53% wanted to go into private group practice.

21.   Trauner, "From Benevolence to Negotiation," 163. For HIP, David R. Hyde and Payson Wolff, "The American Medical Association: Power, Purpose and Politics in Organized Medicine," *Yale Law Review* 63:937 (May 1954), 994–996. In 1944 Garfield told reformers in New York that HIP would fail because it was a mixed closed panel (physicians employed only in the plan) and open panel (physicians may also have outside patients). Also, facilities were owned by outsiders under Blue Cross. Garfield, "Report on Trip to New York RE: Mayor La Guardia's Health Plan," 9 June 1944, carton 37, Henry J. Kaiser Papers, Bancroft Library, University of California, Berkeley [hereafter HJK Papers]. For the UMW, Joel T. Boone, *A Medical Survey of the Bituminous-Coal Industry: Report of the Coal Mines Administration* (Washington, D.C.: Department of the Interior, 1947), 119, in United Mine Workers of America Health and Retirement Funds Archives, West Virginia Collection, University of West Virginia, Morgantown, "The

Boone Report," Box 1 of 1 (hereafter UMWA Archives). A large influx of federal government workers came to Kaiser after the 1959 passage of the Federal Employees Health Benefits Act. Nygren and Childs, *Federal Employees' Health Benefits Program*, 2.

22. For the importance of localism in the AMA constitution of 1901, the early twentieth-century quest for regulation of the medical profession, and competition with other interests: Ronald L. Numbers, *Almost Persuaded: American Physicians and Compulsory Health Insurance, 1912–1920* (Baltimore: Johns Hopkins University Press, 1978), 4, 9, 27–28, 67. For a summary of depression-era economic difficulties and final acceptance by the AMA of voluntary health insurance, see Numbers, "The Third Party: Health Insurance in America," in Judith Walzer Leavitt and Ronald L. Numbers, eds., *Sickness and Health in America: Readings in the History of Medicine and Public Health* (Madison: University of Wisconsin Press, 1985), 236–237. Numbers also notes that the first multiple hospital association to form after the 1929 Baylor plan in creating Blue Cross was in Sacramento in 1932; the California Physicians' Service in 1939 was the first state medical service plan in the formation of Blue Shield.

23. Incomes of small-town doctors declined 17% from 1929 to 1932, with average income for a third of U.S. physicians under $2,300. Committee on the Costs of Medical Care (CCMC), *Medical Care for the American People; The Final Report of the Committee on the Costs of Medical Care, adopted October 31, 1932* (Chicago: University of Chicago Press, 1932), 22–24, 44–46. The California Medical Economic Survey in 1934 reported that the median net income of physicians in the state dropped from $6,000 to $2,800 during the same period. In San Francisco, with a historic oversupply of physicians, doctors' incomes were near those of skilled laborers. See Trauner, "From Benevolence to Negotiation," 142–146, 186. By 1940 Garfield's associates at Grand Coulee had a yearly average salary of about $5,500, with no overhead and only $10 a month for housing. From a ledger sheet titled "Employee's Salaries, Mason City Hospital, 1938–1941," photographic collection, Kaiser Permanente Northern California Region, Oakland, California, compliments of Daniel Scannell, director of public affairs. Numbers emphasizes that the oversupply of poorly qualified physicians was the main problem confronted by the AMA in its efforts to regulate quality, quantity, and income in the profession to the benefit of association members. See Numbers, "The Fall and Rise of the American Medical Profession," in Leavitt and Numbers, *Sickness and Health in America*, 191.

24. Trauner, "From Benevolence to Negotiation," 2–7, 142, 147, 165–166.

25. Rickey L. Hendricks, "Liberal Default, Labor Support, and Conservative Neutrality: The Kaiser Permanente Medical Care Program After World War II," *Journal of Policy History*, 1 (1989), 156–180.

26. *New York Times*, 19 January 1943 (clipping, HJK Papers); Berkowitz and Wolff, *Group Health Association*, 49–55. For the commercialization of medicine in California, see Peter N. Grant, "The Struggle for Control of California's Health Care Marketplace" (Ph.D. diss., Harvard University, 1987). For the declining public image of U.S. doctors: John C. Burnham, "American Medicine's Golden Age: What Happened to It?" *Science*, 19 March 1982, 1474–79, see 1476–77. Also, "U.S. Medicine in Transition," *Science*, December 1944, 156–93.

27. In 1941 the average U.S. doctor earned $5,179, but half netted less than $3,912, and under 1% had a yearly income of $10,000. Permanente doctors received a minimum of $4,800 a year with top salaries of $24,000, and no overhead. Kaiser shipyard workers were well paid by contemporary standards, $61 a week and a gross annual income of $3,172. Sidney R. Garfield, "First Annual Report of the Permanente Foundation Hospitals" (n.d., but c. 1943), carton 330; R. H. Gillespie to E. E. Trefethen, Jr., 6 October 1943, carton 22, HJK Papers. Also, Trauner, "From Benevolence to Negotiation," 6–8, 223–224 (tables 29, 30). Trauner argues that the historic oversupply of physicians in San Francisco and low monthly incomes of public health doctors, comparable to skilled laborers, explain the conservatism of the profession in opposing prepaid group health plans.

1 Reclamation and Health in the Arid West

1. Mark S. Foster, *Henry J. Kaiser: Builder in the Modern American West* (Austin: University of Texas Press, 1989), 30–37.

2. Mumford quoted in Peter Hall, *Cities of Tomorrow: An Intellectual History of Urban Planning and Design in the Twentieth Century* (Oxford: Basil Blackwell, 1988), 152. Daniel M. Fox discusses the intersection of utopian thought, urban planning, and health care in *Health Policies, Health Politics,* 15–20.

3. Franklin D. Roosevelt's support of public power and a greatly increased arable land base for U.S. farmers prompted completion of four massive reclamation projects: the Central Valley project in California, the Colorado River project and Hoover Dam, Grand Coulee Dam in the Columbia River Basin, and the Colorado–Big Thompson project, the only one in which Kaiser was not involved. These projects transformed the semiarid western landscape in the 1930s into productive farmlands that comprised one-third of the total irrigated farm acreage west of the 98th meridian. About 125,000 new family farms and an equal number of suburban homes sprang up in the reclamation areas. Gerald D. Nash, *The American West in the Twentieth Century: A Short History of an Urban Oasis* (Albuquerque: University of New Mexico Press, 1977), 142, 158–159; George Petit, *So Hoover Dam Was Built* (Berkeley: University of California Press, 1935), 21–26.

4. Doyce B. Nunis, Jr., ed., *Men. Medicine, and Water: The Building of the Los Angeles Aqueduct, 1908–1918; A Physician's Recollections by Raymond G. Taylor, MD* (Los Angeles: Friends of the Los Angeles County Medical Association Library and Los Angeles Department of Water and Power, 1982), 15, 163.

5. Derickson, *Workers' Health, Workers' Democracy,* x–xiii, 192–193; Arthur S. Link, *Woodrow Wilson and the Progressive Era, 1910–1917* (New York: Harper & Row, 1954), 228–229, 236; Robert H. Zeiger, *American Workers, American Unions, 1920–1985* (Baltimore: Johns Hopkins University Press, 1986), 22–23.

6. First quote from Cornelius Cochrane, "Meeting a Compensation Medical Problem," *American Labor Legislation Review* 20 (December 1930): 433–435. Second quote from American Medical Association, *Organized*

Payments of Medical Services: A Report Prepared by the Bureau of Medical Economics, American Medical Association (Chicago: AMA, 1939), 150.

7. Schwartz, "Early History of Prepaid Plans," 457– 464.

8. Michael R. Grey, "Poverty, Politics, and Health: The Farm Security Administration Medical Care Program, 1935–1945," *Journal of the History of Medicine and Allied Sciences* 44 (1989), 324.

9. CCMC, *Medical Care for the American People*, 22–24, 44–46; quote, 24. About 22% of those salaried netted between $3,000 and $4,000 a year, while the income peak of the GP was between $1,000 and $2,000 for 17%; one-third of U.S. physicians had a net income of less than $2,300 a year. In California one-third earned less then $2,000 in 1933; one-half less than $3,000. Most U.S. families had incomes under $2,000 at this time with only a small percentage of $4,000 or more. Gross physician income averaged $9,000, but about 40% went for professional expenses. California figures from Grant, "California's Health Care Marketplace," 142.

10. Fox, *Health Policies, Health Politics*, ix, 15–20.

11. CCMC, *Medical Care for the American People*, 154–155.

12. The National Institutes of Health budget grew from $180,000 in 1945 to $46.3 million in 1950, about one-third to extramural grants. Total national expenditures for research rose from about $18 million to $181 million between 1941 and 1951. Starr, *Social Transformation of American Medicine*, 342–343.

13. The classic works are Vogel, *Invention of the Modern Hospital*; Rosner, *A Once Charitable Enterprise*; Rosenberg, *The Care of Strangers*. Talcott Parsons, "Social Change and Medical Organization in the United States: A Sociological Perspective," *Annals of the Academy of Political and Social Science* 346 (March 1963), 21–33. A good critique of the Parsons model is Bryan S. Turner, *Medical Power and Social Knowledge* (London: Sage, 1987), 39–58.

14. Joseph H. Garbarino, *Health Plans and Collective Bargaining* (Berkeley: University of California Press, 1960), 88–89; Margaret Greenfield, *Meeting the Costs of Health Care: The Bay Area Experience and the National Issues* (Berkeley: Institute of Government Studies, University of California, 1972), 11–12, 144; Odin W. Anderson, *Blue Cross Since 1929: Accountability and the Public Trust* (Cambridge, Mass.: Ballinger, 1975), 37–38.

15. Starr, *Social Transformation of American Medicine*, 305–306.

16. Mary Ross, "The Case of the Ross-Loos Clinic," *Survey Graphic* 24:6(June 1935), 302–303; AMA, *Organized Payments for Medical Services*, 132–135.

17. AMA, *Organized Payments for Medical Services*, 134–135.

18. CCMC, *Medical Care for the American People*, 118. Census figures for 1930 estimated from: U.S. Department of Commerce, Bureau of the Census, *Historical Statistics of the United States, Colonial Times to 1970*, part I (Washington, D.C.: U.S. Government Printing Office, 1975), 139, 143, 145 [hereafter *Historical Statistics*].

19. Schwartz, "Early History of Prepaid Plans," 457–464; Washington State Medical Society Committee on Economics, Report of the Committee of Seven, *Northwest Medicine* 31 (1932), 199–203.

20. Morris F. Collen, M.D., "History of the Kaiser Permanente Medical Care Program," an oral history conducted in 1986 by Sally Smith Hughes, Regional Oral History Office, Bancroft Library, University of California, Berkeley, 1988, 9–14. (Henceforth, citations will include interviewer and date on the first reference to an interviewee, Bancroft ROHO history.)

21. CCMC, *Medical Care for the American People*, 22–24; Trauner, "From Benevolence to Negotiation," 224 (table 30).

22. Paul de Kruif, *Kaiser Wakes the Doctors* (New York: Harcourt Brace, 1943), 24–26.

23. CCMC [Minority Report], *Medical Care for the American People*, 156; R. G. Leland, *JAMA* 98(5 March 1932), 805–815.

24. For an overview of the class aspects of the compensation movement in the early twentieth century, Anthony Bale, "America's First Compensation Crisis: Conflict over the Value and Meaning of Workplace Injuries under the Employers' Liability System," *Dying For Work: Workers' Safety and Health in Twentieth-Century America* (Bloomington: Indiana University Press, 1989), 37 (statistics).

25. Theodore White, "Building the Big Dam," *Harper's Magazine*, June 1935, 115; *Report on Hoover Dam Project and Present Status* (Associated General Contractors, December 1931), 68; this report was sponsored by Six Companies when Harold Ickes, secretary of the interior, threatened to fine for overtime violations. Henry J. Kaiser [hereafter HJK] had bound copies sent out, one to Ickes. Petit, *Hoover Dam*, 21–26.

26. Joseph E. Stevens, *Hoover Dam: An American Adventure* (Norman: University of Oklahoma Press, 1988), 62.

27. Ibid., 66–69.

28. Ibid., 69.

29. Minutes, vol. 1, 14 August 1931, Six Companies Records, Bancroft Library, University of California, Berkeley [hereafter Six Companies Records]; quote from New York *New Leader*, 15 August 1931; *San Francisco News*, 26 May 1931; *Information Service* of New York City, 17 October 1931, in Scrapbooks, Six Companies Records; Stevens, *Hoover Dam*, 74–78.

30. Stevens, *Hoover Dam*, 55–64, 288n.

31. *Report on Hoover Dam*, 69.

32. Stevens, *Hoover Dam*, 101.

33. Ibid., 206–214.

34. Ibid, 101.

35. Minutes, vol. 2, 13 August 1932; HJK to Kahn, Department of Interior, Office of the Secretary, Central Classified File, 1907–1936, 3 August 1932, Record Group [hereafter RG] 48, National Archives, Washington, D.C. [hereafter NA].

36. Congressional Hearings, H.R., vol. 632, 28 April 1932, 59–60.

37. Stevens, *Hoover Dam*, 138.

38. Minutes, vol. 1, 18 May 1931, and vol. 2, 18 March 1933; *San Francisco News*, 2 February 1932: Scrapbooks, Six Companies Records.

39. de Kruif, *Kaiser Wakes the Doctors*, 25–26.

40. Cecil C. Cutting, M.D., "Kaiser-Permanente Program History—Presentation for Kaiser-Permanente Executive Program," 15 July 1983, final draft, 5.

41. "Henry J's Proudest Achievement: Kaiser," *Oakland Tribune*, 28 February 1971, 18-X.

42. Nunis, *Men, Medicine and Water*, 153.

43. Raymond M. Kay taped interview by Mark S. Foster, 4 April 1984.

44. Sidney R. Garfield interview by Mark S. Foster, 16 January 1984. Garfield died in February 1985.

45. de Kruif, *Kaiser Wakes the Doctors*, 31–44.

46.   The contract was for Garfield "to furnish certain medical, hospital and health facilities for the benefit of this company's employees employed by it in connection with a contract with the United States of America for the construction of Parker Dam." Work on the dam was interrupted by a large legal blunder. The government neglected to get congressional authorization for the project and the Supreme Court ruled in *U.S. v. Arizona* that work cease until this "oversight" was rectified. Six Companies collected damages of $240,000 from the government for a four-month work stoppage and in turn reimbursed Garfield for $2,350 in losses. Minutes, vol. 2, 28 August 1935, Six Companies Records.

47.   de Kruif, *Kaiser Wakes the Doctors*, 43–49.

48.   Contract and CIO flyer, Box 487; Construction Engineer to Chief Engineer, 17 April 1937, and other documents and records of the Bureau of Reclamation [hereafter BOR], Box 493, RG 115, Office of the Chief Engineer, General Correspondence—Straights, file 31-M, National Archives, Denver Branch [hereafter NA, Denver]; *Engineering News-Record* 115 (15 July 1937), and 119 (5 August 1937), 206.

49.   Howard Kimeldorf, *Reds or Rackets? The Making of Radical and Conservative Unions on the Waterfront* (Berkeley: University of California Press, 1988), 19–35; Nash, *American West*, 70–73. With the deteriorating position of labor during the post–World War I reactionism dubbed the "Red Scare," mainstream unionists such as John L. Lewis and Samuel Gompers reacted against labor's left wing. So did the courts, which issued the broadest strike injunctions in history, invalidated minimum wage laws, and struck down the labor safeguards in the 1914 Clayton Act. By 1923, when immigration restriction stemmed the influx of the more radical foreign workers, membership in labor organizations declined by one million to 3,780,000. The strength of the movement was not revitalized until the depression and New Deal of the 1930s. See David Brody, *Workers in Industrial America: Essays on the Twentieth Century Struggle* (New York: Oxford University Press, 1980), pp. 24–46.

50.   Harre W. Demoro, "Strike of '34 Put Harry Bridges in Labor's Vanguard," *San Francisco Chronicle*, 31 March 1990, A4.

51.   Nash, *American West*, 142, 158–59; Petit, *Hoover Dam*, 21–26.

52.   *Facts About Henry J. Kaiser* (Oakland: Kaiser Co., 16 September 1946), 49. Members of Consolidated Builders, Inc., were Henry J. Kaiser Co. (sponsor and manager), Kaiser Co., Pacific Bridge Co., MacDonald and Kahn, Inc., Utah Construction Co., Morrison-Knudson Co., Inc., J. F. Shea, Inc., General Construction Co., and Mason-Walsh-Atkinson-Kier Co. The nearly $41 million project, completed in December 1942, involved pouring approximately 5,500,000 cubic yards of mass cement.

53.   Quoted in Richard C. Neuberger, "The Biggest Thing on Earth: Grand Coulee Dam," *Harper's Magazine*, February 1954, 255. Richard Lowitt, *The New Deal and the West* (Bloomington: Indiana University Press, 1984), 166; Murray Morgan, *The Dam* (New York: Viking, 1954), 67–68. F. J. Sharkey, "Schools in the Grand Coulee Dam Area," unpublished report to Chief Engineer Frank A. Banks, 16 March 1936, BOR Office of the Chief Engineer.

54.   Chief Engineer to Construction Engineer, 30 September 1938; Acting Supervising Engineer to Chief Engineer, 10 July 1939; Engineer to Chief Engineer, 23 November 1942, all in Box 442, RG 115, General Correspondence—Engineering, file 791-H, NA, Denver; *Engineering News-Rec-*

ord, 115 (1 August 1935), 145, and 117 (10 September 1936), 364. It was envisioned that Coulee Dam and Mason City would eventually be incorporated on the model of Boulder City. Lowitt, *New Deal and the West*, has the two towns reversed.

55. This also is Richard Lowitt's interpretation in *New Deal and the West*, 226; Kaiser biographer Mark S. Foster disagrees that Henry J. Kaiser was launched by the New Deal. He suggests a similar interpretation in "Giant of the West" but gives Kaiser credit for individual initiative and the ability to manipulate the relationship between the corporation and the federal government to advantage. See "Giant of the West: Henry J. Kaiser and Regional Industrialization, 1930–1950, *Business History Review* 59:1 (Spring 1985).

56. Contract and CIO flyer, Box 487; Construction Engineer to Chief Engineer, 17 April 1937, and other documents and records of the BOR, Box 493, RG 115, Office of the Chief Engineer, General Correspondence—Straights, file 31-M, NA, Denver; *Engineering News-Record* 115 (15 July 1937), and 119 (5 August 1937), 206.

57. Schwartz, "Early History of Prepaid Plans," 457–462.

58. Garfield interview by Foster, 6 January 1984.

59. Ibid.; E. R. Ordway interview by Mark S. Foster, 13 January 1984.

60. De Kruif, *Kaiser Wakes the Doctors*, 50.

61. Quotes from *Kaiser 50th Anniversary Book*, "The Hospital in the Desert," 7–8, carton 295, HJK Papers; de Kruif, *Kaiser Wakes the Doctors*, 50–55.

62. DeKruif, *Kaiser Wakes the Doctors*, 54–55; Cecil C. Cutting interview by Malca Chall, 1986, Bancroft ROHO history, 7–8; Cecil C. Cutting interview by Mark S. Foster, 12 January 1984, Oakland, California.

63. Sidney R. Garfield interview by Mimi Stein, 17 February 1982, unedited draft, 17.

64. Ibid.; Cutting, "Kaiser-Permanente Program History," 8; de Kruif, *Kaiser Wakes the Doctors*, 54–55.

65. Sample payroll check, BOR, Box 442, RG 115, Office of the Chief Engineer, General Correspondence—Engineering, file 791-H, NA, Denver. By a wage agreement with MWAK following the threatened strikes in 1937, the AFL International and Local agreements approved a job classification schedule with 135 categories and an hourly wage range of $0.65 for unskilled to $1.65 for highly skilled labor. Highest paid were divers at $3.20 an hour; next highest, $1.65 for line workers and hoist operators. The CIO did not sign the contract. Ibid., Box 487 General Correspondence—Straights, file 31-M.

66. Cutting, "Kaiser-Permanente Program History," 9.

67. de Kruif, *Kaiser Wakes the Doctors*, 56–57. Garfield interview by Stein, 22.

68. Garfield interview by Stein, 22; Cutting, "Kaiser-Permanente Program History," 9.

69. de Kruif, *Kaiser Wakes the Doctors*, 59.

70. Garfield interview by Stein, 23–24; *Kaiser 50th Anniversary Book*, 8; de Kruif, *Kaiser Wakes the Doctors*, 59–60.

71. Garfield interview by Foster.

72. Cutting, Bancroft ROHO history, 7; Eugene E. Trefethen interview by Malca Chall, 1986, ibid., 6, 17; Ernest W. Saward interview by Sally Smith Hughes, 1986, ibid., 56.

73. Supervising Engineer to Commissioner, 10 July 1942, BOR, Box 461, RG 115, Office of the Chief Engineer, General Correspondence, file 796-F, NA, Denver.

74. John C. Page, Commissioner BOR, to Secretary of Interior, 29 June 1940; Northwest Defense Council Resolutions, 24 July 1940; Supervising Engineer to Commissioner, 16 August 1940, all in BOR, Box 414, RG 115, Office of the Chief Engineer, General Correspondence—Engineering, file 791, NA, Denver.

75. AMA, *Organized Payments of Medical Services*, 143.

76. Morris Fishbein, "American Medicine and the National Health Plan," *New England Journal of Medicine*, 23 March 1939, 502.

77. The Bay Area was 38% union by 1960. Carl T. Hall, "San Francisco Has Changed Since Harry's Day," San Francisco *Chronicle*, 31 March 1990, Business Section, 1. For other population estimates, *Historical Statistics*, 14, 82, 131, 140, 177. On national statistics, Raymond Munts, *Bargaining For Health: Labor Unions, Health Insurance, and Medical Care* (Madison: University of Wisconsin Press, 1967), 6–7, 249n; CCMC, *Medical Care for the American People*, 118. On practitioners' status, Trauner, "From Benevolence to Negotiation," 2–3, 142, 147, 165–166.

2   Shipyard Communities and Occupational Health

1. Gerald D. Nash introduces the regional image of "urban oases" in *The Short History of an Urban Oasis*, 2d ed. (Albuquerque: University of New Mexico Press, 1977). A recent overview of urban transformation in Oakland and Richmond is: Marilynn S. Johnson, "Urban Arsenals: War Housing and Social Change in Richmond and Oakland, California, 1941–1945," *Pacific Historical Review*, 60:3, 283–308. For social change from a feminist perspective in Portland and Vancouver: Amy Kesselman, *Fleeting Opportunities: Women Shipyard Workers in Portland and Vancouver During World War II and Reconversion* (Albany: State University of New York, 1990).

2. Mel Scott, *The San Francisco Bay Area; A Metropolis in Perspective*, 2d ed. (Berkeley: University of California Press, 1985), 221, 244–248; Gerald D. Nash, *The American West Transformed: The Impact of the Second World War* (Bloomington: Indiana University Press, 1985), 56–59, 75–76. *Historical Statistics*, 24–37; Johnson, "Urban Arsenals," 283–287.

3. Collen, Bancroft ROHO history, 10, 13–14, 17–24; also, Sally Smith Hughes, "Interview History," in Collen, ibid., vi–vii.

4. Joel D. Howell, "Hearts and Minds: The Invention and Transformation of American Cardiology," in Russell C. Maulitz and Diana E. Long, eds., *Grand Rounds: One Hundred Years of Internal Medicine* (Philadelphia: University of Pennsylvania Press, 1988), 248, 250–251, 258–260. Stevens, *In Sickness and In Wealth*, 203–204, 397n13, 399n60.

5. Figures in Starr, *Social Transformation of American Medicine*, 358–359.

6. *Facts About Henry J. Kaiser*, 18, 47; "The Earthmovers II," *Fortune* September 1943, 17–19; Alyce M. Kramer, "The Story of the Richmond Shipyards," n.d., unpublished typescript, carton 330, HJK Papers. Foster, *Henry J. Kaiser* and "Giant of the West," 1–23.

7. Ibid.

8. Scott, *San Francisco Bay Area*, 88–91, 217, 248–257; Nash, *American West Transformed*, 75–76; William H. Harris, "Federal Intervention in Union Discrimination: FEPC and West Coast Shipyards During World War II," *Labor History* 22:3 (Summer 1981), 326.

9. Federal Security Agency (FSA) report, "Population Shifts in Richmond Shipbuilding Area," n.d., but c. summer 1943, carton 186, HJK Papers; Kramer, "Story of the Richmond Shipyards"; "Fact Sheet on Wartime Richmond," carton 330, HJK Papers. Nash, *American West Transformed*, 56–59, 75–76.

10. *Fortune* magazine reported that Kaiser was "anxious to avoid jurisdictional battles with the CIO," and particularly with Harry Bridges's Longshoremen. "After the Battle; Out of the Bloody Past Labor Unions and Employers' Associations Have Worked a Hopeful Pattern of Agreement," *Fortune*, February 1945, 179, quote on 326; de Kruif, *Kaiser Wakes the Doctors*, 70–72.

11. Report to B. K. Ogden, Director, Division of Insurance, USMC, for A. B. Ordway, Vice-president Richmond Shipyards, 31 August 1943, "Richmond Shipyards Industrial Medical and Hospital Facilities," carton 330, HJK Papers; *Facts About Henry J. Kaiser*, "Kaiser Enterprise At War," 29–31.

12. de Kruif, *Kaiser Wakes the Doctors*, 70–71; report, Kaiser Company, Inc., Vancouver Yard, "Report on Labor Utilization," 8 February 1944, carton 329, HJK Papers.

13. Nash, *American West Transformed*, 56–59, 75–76.

14. FSA, "Population Shifts"; Katherine Hamill, "Richmond Took a Beating," 18 December 1944, typescript for *Fortune*, carton 330, HJK Papers; photo captions, Kaiser Photographs, Richmond Shipyards, Housing, 1983.19, Bancroft Library, University of California, Berkeley.

15. Carl Abbott, "Planning for the Home Front in Seattle and Portland, 1900–1945," in Roger Lotchin, ed., *The Martial Metropolis: U.S. Cities in War and Peace* (New York: Praeger, 1984), 166–172; *Bo's'n's Whistle*, n.v. (27 September 1942), 20.

16. D. D. Lester Lynch, "Vanport, Oregon's Second City," *Western Construction News*, 18 (August 1943), 351–354.

17. *Bo's'n's Whistle* 2:17(10 September 1942), 1; *Bo's'n's Whistle* 3:10(20 May 1943), 8.

18. E. Kimbark MacColl, *The Growth of a City: Power and Politics in Portland, Oregon, 1915–1950* (Portland: Georgian Press, 1979), 578; Abbott, "Planning for the Home Front," 181; Nash, *American West Transformed*, 77–78. Individualism and urban aesthetics would have another chance in the Portland-Vancouver area. Vanport was washed away in a flood in 1948. According to Nash the war had little lasting impact on the area.

19. Garfield interview by Stein, 33–39.

20. Garfield, "First Annual Report"; Cutting interview by Foster.

21. Garfield interview by Stein, 5–6, 34. For a thumbnail sketch of Giannini see Nash, *American West Transformed*, 33–34; de Kruif, *Kaiser Wakes the Doctors*, 26–27.

22. Garfield interview by Foster; Scott Fleming, "Kaiser Permanente Overview" (Oakland: Kaiser Foundation Health Plan, 1 May 1986).

23. Garfield interview by Stein, 22–27.

24. *Facts About Henry J. Kaiser*, 29–30; FSA, "Population Shifts"; de Kruif, *Kaiser Wakes the Doctors*, 96–97.

25. FSA, "Population Shifts"; de Kruif, *Kaiser Wakes the Doctors*, 96–97.

26. Garfield interview by Stein, 33–39; *Bo's'n's Whistle* 2:17(10 September 1942).

27. FSA, "Population Shifts"; Hamill, "Richmond Took a Beating"; photo captions, Kaiser Photographs, Richmond Shipyards, Housing, 1983.19, Bancroft Library, University of California, Berkeley; *Facts About Henry J. Kaiser*, "Kaiser Enterprise At War," 29–31; FSA, Office of Defense, Health and Welfare Services, "Inspection of Trailer Camps and Shack Developments in the Unincorporated Area Surrounding Richmond, California," n.d., but c. April 1943, carton 186, HJK Papers.

28. Fact Sheet on Wartime Richmond, excerpted from Katherine Hamill, "Richmond Took a Beating," 18 December 1944, typescript for *Fortune*, February 1945, carton 330, HJK Papers; HJK to Ralph Paine and K. Hamill, 26 December 1944, carton 25, HJK Papers; Philip S. Foner, *Women and the American Labor Movement* (New York: Macmillan, 1982), 354–355.

29. Memo, Erik Holtemann to HJK, 26 August 1942, carton 330, HJK Papers.

30. "To Our Employees," cover letter signed by Clay Bedford on pamphlet entitled "A Health Plan for the Employees of the Richmond Shipyard," n.d., c. 1942, carton 309, HJK Papers.

31. Algie Martin Simons and Nathan Sinai, *The Way of Health Insurance* (Chicago: University of Chicago Press, 1932), 15–17, 206–207.

32. See Turner, *Medical Power and Social Knowledge*, 39–58; also, N. Jewson, "The Disappearance of the Sick Man from Medical Cosmology, 1770–1870," *Sociology* 10 (1976), 225–244.

33. Report by L. L. Reise, "The Changes in Population and Medical Care Facilities in Vancouver . . . vs. Portland Oregon," December 1943, carton 183, HJK Papers.

34. Ibid.

35. Kramer, "Story of the Richmond Shipyards."

36. Nash, *American West Transformed*, 56–59, 75–76.

37. Jean Johnson (Hiring Hall) to James C. Egan, 7 January 1943, and Johnson to Egan, 9 March 1943, "Men Arriving from the East on Contract Who Did Not Sign on Payroll through 31 January 1943," carton 23, HJK Papers; Kramer, "Story of the Richmond Shipyards."

38. Ibid.; Allan M. Brandt, *No Magic Bullet: A Social History of Venereal Disease in the United States Since 1880*, rev. ed. (New York: Oxford University Press, 1987), 169.

39. Reise, "Changes in Population."

40. Brandt, *No Magic Bullet*, 169; E. E. Trefethen, Jr., to Garfield, 1 November 1943; mimeo, "Annual Report on Research and Medical Care Programs for the Permanente Foundation for 1944, and Forecast for 1945," carton 309, HJK Papers. Cutting interview by Foster; Morris F. Collen, M.D., "The Treatment of Pneumococcic Pneumonia With Penicillin and Sulfadiazine," *California Medicine* 66:2, 62–65; Collen, "Problems in the Treatment of Viral Pneumonia," *Permanente Foundation Medical Bulletin* 10:1–4 (August 1952), 237.

41. Johnson to Egan, 9 March 1943, carton 23, HJK Papers; Nash, *American West Transformed*, 89–91. On the West's black population, see Nash, 89–91.

42. Harris, "Federal Intervention in Union Discrimination," 334–338; "Percentage of Negroes to Total Work Force in the Three Kaiser Yards,

Portland and Vancouver," Fair Employment Practices Commission (FEPC) Papers, Box 321-C, RG 228, NA.

43. Johnson, "Urban Arsenals" 304–307 (Welfare Council quote, 306).

44. Ibid.

45. Harris, "Federal Intervention in Union Discrimination," 341–342. Harris's findings are based on the FEPC West Coast Hearings, Portland, FEPC HQ Recs., Rolls 13, 14, 1943. For Edgar Kaiser's personal involvement: George M. Johnson, Asst. Exec. Sec., FEPC, to Edgar Kaiser [hereafter EFK], 30 June 1943; Malcolm Ross, FEPC Chairman to EFK, 28 December 1943, FEPC Papers, Box 46, RG 228, NA. EFK to HJK, 12 July 1944, carton 25, HJK Papers.

46. "Percentage of Negroes." For Edgar Kaiser's personal involvement see Edgar Kaiser to HJK, 12 July 1944, carton 25, HJK Papers; George M. Johnson, Asst. Exec. Sec., FEPC, to EFK, 30 June 1943; Malcolm Ross, FEPC chair, to EFK, 28 December 1943; Cornelius Golightly to John A. Davis, 15 August 1944, FEPC Papers, Box 46, RG 228, NA; MacColl, *Growth of a City*, 583–596; Fleming, "Kaiser Permanente Overview," 6. "Permanente Health Plan Recommended by Oakland Council for Future Contracts," ILWU *Dispatcher* 3:12(15 June 1945), 14.

47. Reise, "Changes in Population"; Senate Special Committee for Defense Contracts, *Investigation of National Defense Program, 30 July 1942*, 4146–4147.

48. Memo, Charles H. Day to C. P. Bedford, 26 April 1943, carton 330, HJK Papers. Memo from Drs. C. C. Cutting and L. L. Reise, April 1943, carton 183, HJK Papers.

49. Kramer, "Story of the Richmond Shipyards"; Kaiser testimony, Senate, Special Committee Investigating the National Defense Program, *Hearings, 9 March 1943*, 725; *Bo's'n's Whistle*, n.v. (19 August 1943), 2; *Bo's'n's Whistle* 4:1(14 January 1944), 5; Nash, *American West Transformed*, 40–41. *Bo's'n's Whistle*, n.v. (19 August 1943), 2.

50. Eleanor Roosevelt to Admiral Land, 9 June 1943, U.S. Maritime Commission Records, Box 3, RG178, E. S. Land, Misc. Files, NA; Mary Kinnear, *Daughters of Time: Women in the Western Tradition* (Ann Arbor: University of Michigan Press, 1982), 170–171. Though the Kaiser company was not responsible for the existence of child care centers in Richmond, in Portland-Vancouver the company established two such centers staffed by 100 teachers, ten registered nurses, a medical consultant, and five child nutritionists. Attendance at each was about 275 daily in 1944. See *Facts About Henry J. Kaiser*, 31; Mildred Cutting to Anne Gould, 17 April 1947, carton 35, HJK Papers.

51. Foner, *Women and the American Labor Movement*, 355.

52. Kesselman, *Fleeting Opportunities*, 68–69.

53. Ibid., 74–75.

54. Ibid., 76–77.

55. Ibid., 75–77 (quote, 75).

56. Robert D. Lasker to HJK, 27 April 1943, carton 176; Booklet, "A Health Plan for the Employees of the Richmond Shipyards," n.d., c. 1942, carton 309, HJK Papers; Report by L. L. Reise attached to "Changes in Population." For addition of maternity benefits in 1944, see booklet, "Group Hospital and Surgical Insurance," offered by Kaiser affiliates, June 1944, carton 330, HJK Papers.

57. Quote is from "Women in Shipbuilding: A Graphic Portrayal of the First Six Months Experience of Women Employed in the Kaiser Shipyards" (Oakland: Kaiser Co. Inc., 1 January 1943), carton 330, HJK Papers. de Kruif, *Kaiser Wakes the Doctors*, 92–93; Cutting, "Kaiser-Permanente Program History." Senate Committee on Education and Labor, 77th Congress, 2d Sess., Hearings on S. Res. 291, Pt. 2, pp. 325–347, 2–3 November 1942 (reprinted in *JAMA*, 120 [21 November 1942], 940) [hereafter Hearings on S. Res. 291].

58. Hamill, "Richmond Took a Beating," 268.

59. James A. Routh to Garfield, 12 July 1944, attached to "Analysis of Proposed Health Plan for Harbor Gate Residents," carton 330; Garfield to "Boss," 14 March 1944, carton 175, HJK Papers.

60. Memo, T. T. Inch to Garfield, 13 September 1945, carton 183; mimeo, "Origin and Development of the Principles of the Kaiser Health Plan," n.d., c. 1945, carton 330, HJK Papers.

61. *Fore n' Aft*, 30 July 1942 and 20 August 1942, carton 309, HJK Papers. Garfield, "Health Plan Principles," 338.

62. *Facts About Henry J. Kaiser*, "Kaiser Enterprises at War," 29–31. Most of the Kaiser medical land and buildings were mortgaged to the Bank of America. Mimeo, "Kaiser Foundation Balance Sheet—A Summary of Existing Facilities, Recorded Cost of Expansion Program to October 31, 1953," carton 89, HJK Papers.

63. Garfield to Charles Kramer (Pepper Committee, Union Health Subcommittee), 23 November 1945, carton 330; chart, c. 1956, "Membership Growth," 1943–55, carton 124; table, "Health Plan Membership for Selected Years," carton 339, HJK Papers. Fleming, "Kaiser-Permanente Program History," 6–7.

64. Garfield interview by Foster.

65. Starr, *Social Transformation of American Medicine*, 311–312, 325; Nelson Lichtenstein, *Labor's War At Home: The CIO in World War II* (Cambridge: Cambridge University Press, 1982), 240; Garbarino, *Health Plans and Collective Bargaining*, 18–20; *JAMA*, special edition, part 1, 17 January 1959, 56; Anderson, *Blue Cross Since 1929*, 45; Michael Davis, *Medical Care for Tomorrow* (New York: Harper Bros., 1955), 231–232; Anne R. Somers, ed., *The Kaiser Permanente Medical Care Program: One Valid Solution to the Problem of Health Care Delivery in the United States, Proceedings of a Symposium in Oakland, California* (New York: Commonwealth Fund, 1971), 199. At the end of 1947 only 3% of 32,000 group members in the Kaiser Health Plan in the San Francisco Bay Area had employer payment of benefits; by mid-1955 this number had risen to 33% of 226,000 group members. Total membership in northern California in 1955 was 301,671.

66. "Central Labor Council Endorses Permanente Health Plan," *East Bay Labor Journal* 20:15(8 February 1946), p. 1; general release by the Permanente Metals Corp., n.d., but c. late 1945, carton 183, HJK Papers; Kaiser to Senator James E. Murray, Committee on Labor and Public Welfare, U.S. Senate, 27 June 1949, read into *Congressional Record* by Murray, carton 45, HJK Papers.

67. "Health Plan Opened to Bay Unions," ILWU *Dispatcher* 3:11(1 June 1945), 12; "Permanente Health Plan Recommended by Oakland Council for Future Contracts," ibid. 3:12 (July 1945), 14; "Longshoremen Sign Up for Permanente Health Plan," ibid. 3:23 (November 1945), 5.

68. Kimeldorf, *Reds or Rackets?*, 144–151.

69. Zeiger, *American Workers, American Unions*, 124–125; Clifford H. Keene, M.D., speech to U.S. Steelworkers convention, 18 September 1954, carton 103, HJK Papers; Fleming, "Kaiser-Permanente Program History," 18; Avram Yedidia, an interview conducted in 1985 by Ora Huth, Bancroft ROHO history, 53–54.

70. Saward, Bancroft ROHO history, 32–36. Stevens, *In Sickness and In Wealth*, 203–204, 397n13, 399n60.

71. Saward, Bancroft ROHO history, 32–36. Yedidia, Bancroft ROHO history, 31–35.

72. Saward, Bancroft ROHO history, 33; table, "Health Plan Membership for Selected Years," carton 339, HJK Papers.

73. Garfield interview by Foster; Raymond M. Kay, *Historical Review of the Southern California Permanente Medical Group* (Los Angeles: Southern California Permanente Medical Group, 1979), 6–7.

74. Joseph T. DeSilva, "Need a Doctor? A Union Finds A Way," *Nation*, 18 September 1954, 229–230; Yedidia, Bancroft ROHO history, 58, 68; booklet, *The Permanente Health Plan and A Proposal for Los Angeles and San Francisco*, "Representative Health Plan Groups, Bay Area, March 1951" [hereafter "Bay Area Proposal"], carton 87:18, EFK Papers. Kay, *Historical Review*, 6–7; Garfield interview by Foster.

75. Fairley to Liebenson, 4 November 1952; memo, Fairley to ILWU Warehouse and Fish Locals, 19 August 1953; and typescript, report by Percy Moore, Welfare Director, Local 6, 18 April 1955, History Files, Warehouse Welfare Correspondence; memo, "Summary of ILWU-PMA Welfare Plan," History Files, Health Plans, Brochures, 1953–67, all in International Longshoremen's and Warehousemen's Union (ILWU) Library, San Francisco. Total membership figures: table, "Health Plan Membership For Selected Years," carton 339; table 1, "Total Health Plan Membership January 1953–June 1955," carton 117, HJK Papers. Membership itemized by unions by dividing utilization data in table 1 (mimeo, "Kaiser Foundation Health Plan, Southern California Division, Utilization of Facilities by membership through Retail Clerks, Culinary Group, Longshore Groups," 1953–55) by average inpatient and outpatient visits per member in table 5 (mimeo, "Kaiser Foundation Health Plan, Southern California Division, Utilization Statistics, 1953–1955)," carton 132:21, EFK Papers.

76. Computed from membership figures given by Saward in "Documentation of Twenty Years of Operation and Growth of a Prepaid Group Practice Plan," *Medical Care* 6 (May–June 1968), 232–233; interoffice memo, Sam G. Hufford (Regional Manager) to E. E. Trefethen, et al., 2 August 1956, carton 309, HJK Papers.

77. Garbarino, *Health Plans and Collective Bargaining*, 27, 216–217; table, "Kaiser Foundation Health Plan Membership . . . for the Years 1950 to 1963," carton 247, HJK Papers; "Hotel and Bar Workers—12,500 in AF of L to Join Kaiser Plan on April 1," San Francisco *Chronicle*, 8 March 1954, n.p., carton 89, HJK Papers. For membership computation, see note 75.

78. Yedidia, Bancroft ROHO history, 52–57; "Bay Area Proposal."

79. AMA, Commission on Medical Care Plans, "Report," *JAMA*, special edition, part 1, 17 January 1959, 6; "U.S. Medicine in Transition," *Fortune*, December 1944, 156–157, 160, 161–163; Garfield, "Kaiser Co. Makes It Work," 18.

80. HJK to C. E. Wilson, 14 December 1942, carton 22, HJK Papers.

3   The Politics of
National Health

1. Garfield, "Health Plan Principles," 337, 347.
2. Mimeo, "Summary of a Conference between Dr. Cecil C. Cutting and Dr. Harold Fletcher," 10 October 1942, carton 309, HJK Papers.
3. AMA, *Organized Payment of Medical Services*, 181 (quote), 17, 100–102.
4. Anderson, *Blue Cross Since 1929*, 49–50, 54–57; Monte M. Poen, *The Genesis of Medicare* (Columbia: University of Missouri Press, 1979); *Harry S. Truman versus the Medical Lobby*, 29–31; Schwartz, "Early History of Prepaid Plans," 463–475; Also, Grant, "California's Health Care Marketplace," 72–79; "4498 State Doctors Join Medical Aid Unit," San Francisco *Chronicle*, 3 April 1939, 10; J. Philo Nelson to HJK, 4 February 1943, carton 330, HJK Papers. The historic source for the interpretation of state medical society–controlled plans as reactive is Hyde and Wolff, "American Medical Association," 992.
5. Schwartz, "Early History of Prepaid Plans," 463–475; Starr, *Social Transformation of American Medicine*, 325. Lawrence D. Brown also makes this argument in *Politics and Health Care Organization—HMOs as Federal Policy* (Washington, D.C.: Brookings Institution, 1983), 43.
6. Garfield to Frank H. Lahey, 3 November 1942, carton 309, HJK Papers.
7. Trefethen to HJK, 27 November 1943; F. A. Stewart to Mrs. Franklin D. Roosevelt, 17 May 1943; Garfield to Mrs. Roosevelt, 25 May 1943, carton 309, HJK Papers. Garfield interview by Stein, 14–17.
8. Hearings on S. Res. 291, 927–967. Fishbein, editorial, *JAMA*, 120 (14 November 1942), 840–841. Kaiser testimony, Senate, Special Committee Investigating the National Defense Program, *Hearings, 9 March 1943*, 726–727.
9. Kramer, "Story of the Richmond Shipyards." Handwritten note, "Sid" to "Boss," 3 March 1943, carton 19, HJK Papers.
10. Joint Report of Alameda County Medical Association, East Bay Hospital Conference, 15 June 1943, carton 309, HJK Papers. Minutes, Coordinating Committee of Procurement and Assignment Service, 1 November 1943, carton 309, HJK Papers.
11. HJK to C. E. Wilson, 14 December 1943; and "Answers to Questions," undated, carton 22, HJK Papers.
12. FSA, "Population Shifts"; Reise, "Changes in Population." On funding, *Facts About Henry J. Kaiser*, 29–30.
13. Franklin Roosevelt did not support the bill openly, though he privately took credit for the cradle-to-grave insurance concepts being touted by British spokesperson Sir William Beveridge in a U.S. lecture tour. Democrats were divided and Republicans of the 78th Congress were strongest since the 1920s. The demise of many New Deal agencies in mid-1943 when Congress denied funding made political fodder of any further welfare proposals. Nevertheless, Roosevelt was a political opportunist, continuing to express support of national health insurance to William Green of the AFL, and Philip Murray of the CIO. See Poen, *Harry S. Truman*, 29–30. Also Daniel S. Hirshfield, *The Lost Reform: The Campaign for Compulsory Health in*

the United States from 1932–1943 (Cambridge, Mass.: Harvard University Press, 1970).

14. Edward D. Berkowitz, *America's Welfare State from Roosevelt to Reagan* (Baltimore: Johns Hopkins University Press, 1991), 154–157.

15. 317 U.S. 519 (1943). "AMA Loses Fight in Supreme Court in Health Plan; Its Conviction Under Antitrust Law in Cooperative Case Unanimously Upheld," *New York Times*, 19 January 1943; *JAMA*, special edition, 17 January 1959, 6–8; de Kruif, *Kaiser Wakes the Doctors*, 78–87, 123–124. The definitive history of GHA is Berkowitz and Wolff, *Group Health Association*.

16. John C. Burnham, "American Medicine's Golden Age: What Happened to It?" *Science*, 19 March 1982, 1474–1479.

17. Examples of legislative articles in the ILWU *Dispatcher* are: "Questions and Answers on Health Insurance Bills," 3:2(26 January 1945), 12; "Health Plan Opened to Bay Unions," 3:11(1 June 1945), 12; "Ickes, in Sharp Exchange, Backs Murray Health Bill," 4:8(19 April 1946), 16; "Pepper Drafts Omnibus Health Bill for Senate" and "What About Those Promises: Watch out for tricks in the 81st Congress; Truman promised a lot, but . . .", 7:2(21 January 1949), 1. Quotes are from "Medical Profits Go Red, White and Blue," 8:30(October 27, 1949), 5, and "Caucus Raps AMA's Anti-Health Drive," 8:30(27 October 1950), 7.

18. Garbarino, *Health Plans and Collective Bargaining*, 91–93; Poen, *Harry S. Truman*, 29–32, 66–68; Edward Berkowitz and Kim McQuaid, *Creating the Welfare State: The Political Economy of Twentieth-Century Reform* (New York: Praeger, 1980), 129–131. For California health care legislative initiatives see Greenfield, *Meeting the Costs of Health Care*, 144.

19. "Memo on Governor Warren Call on Kaiser on Nationwide Medical Center Program," n.d., carton 92, HJK Papers.

20. Starr, *Social Transformation of American Medicine*, 278–279.

21. Quoted in Poen, *Harry S. Truman*, 148–149. None of the series of Wagner-Murray-Dingell bills proposed between 1943 (as S. 1320) and 1949 (as S. 1679 and H.R. 4312) was radical in its provisions. They structured a national system based on decentralized administration at the local level, with prepaid services based on individual needs and fee-for-service payment to doctors. Poen, *Harry S. Truman*, 170.

22. Starr, *Social Transformation of American Medicine*, 278–279; Poen, *Harry S. Truman*, 29–30; Fox, *Health Policies, Health Politics*, 115; Berkowitz, *America's Welfare State*, 155.

23. AMA, Commission on Medical Care Plans, Report, *JAMA*, special edition, part 1, 17 January 1959, 6; *Historical Statistics*, 9, 177.

24. Berkowitz, *America's Welfare State*, 157–158.

25. Fiorello La Guardia to HJK, 20 May 1944; HJK to La Guardia, 24 January 1945; Paul S. Marrin to Paul F. Cadman, 27 June 1946, carton 37, HJK Papers.

26. Garfield to "Boss," 14 March 1944, carton 175; Garfield, "Paper on Postwar Industrial Health," February 1944, carton 330, and "Report on Trip to New York Re: Mayor La Guardia's Health Plan," 9 June 1944, carton 37, HJK Papers.

27. Letters, *Fortune*, January 1945, 17–18.

28. Kaiser to Mrs. Albert D. Lasker, 21 November 1945, carton 33; Robert F. Wagner to HJK, 7 December 1944; HJK to Wagner, 30 December 1944, carton 30, HJK Papers. Fiorello La Guardia to HJK, 20 May 1944;

HJK to La Guardia, 24 January 1945; Paul S. Marin to Paul F. Cadman, 27 June 1946, carton 37, HJK Papers.

29. Garfield to "Boss," 14 March 1944, carton 175, HJK Papers; Garfield, "Paper on Postwar Industrial Health," carton 330, HJK Papers.

30. HJK to Hon. Henry A. Wallace, 13 March 1945; "A National Medical Plan Based on the Existing Facilities and the Operating Program of the Permanente Foundation"; Trefethen to Paul F. Cadman, 21 March 1945; memo and "Draft of Statement for Pepper Committee," 29 March 1945, carton 189, HJK Papers.

31. Boone, *Medical Survey of the Bituminous-Coal Industry*, 119, UMWA Archives.

32. Webster, *Health Services Since the War*, 41–42; Fox, *Health Policies, Health Politics*, 105, 261.

33. Robert A. Levine, "Rethinking Our Social Strategies," *Public Interest*, Winter 1968, 88; Joseph L. Falkson, *HMOs and the Politics of Health System Reform* (Chicago: Robert J. Brady Co. for American Hospital Association, 1980), 13–15. Garfield to Henry A. Wallace, 28 March 1945, carton 183, HJK Papers.

34. HJK to Senator Claude Pepper, 1 July 1945, carton 47, HJK Papers.

35. Starr, *Social Transformation of American Medicine*, 425; AMA, *Organized Payments of Medical Services*, 150–151.

36. Brody, *Workers in Industrial America*, 190–199.

37. Clifford H. Keene, M.D., "Status of Hospitalization Plans for Willow Run," report, 7 November 1947, HJK Papers (no carton number).

38. Truman quote in Robert J. Donovan, *Conflict and Crisis: The Presidency of Harry S Truman, 1945–1948* (New York: Norton, 1977), 212–218.

39. Fred Grimm, "Coal Miners Struggle for Union's Future," *Miami Herald*, 8 July 1989, 1, 6A; Robert H. Zeiger, *John J. Lewis—Labor Leader* (Boston: Twayne, 1988), 150–179.

40. "Directory of Union-sponsored Health Centers and Medical Service Programs," published by the Committee for the Nation's Health, *Labor Health and Welfare Series*, revised 18 December 1953, carton 103, HJK Papers, listed AFL Medical Service Plan, Philadelphia (1951); Labor Health Institute, St. Louis (1945-Teamsters); Sidney Hillman Health Center, Chicago (1951); Amalgamated Meat Cutters and Butcher Workmen, New York City (three centers); International Ladies Garment Workers Union centers (1913–51) in Los Angeles; Boston and Fall River, Mass.; Minneapolis; Kansas City, Mo.; St. Louis; Newark; New York City; Cleveland; Allentown, Harrisburg, Philadelphia, Wilkes-Barre, Pa.; Dallas and San Antonio, with centers planned for Washington, D.C., and San Francisco.

41. Fairley to Liebenson, 4 November 1952; memo, Fairley to ILWU Warehouse and Fish Locals, 19 August 1953; and typescript, Percy Moore, Welfare Director, Local 6, 18 April 1955, History Files—Warehouse Welfare Correspondence; memo, "Summary of ILWU-PMA Welfare Plan," History Files, Health Plans, Brochures, 1953–67, ILWU Library.

42. E. Richard Weinerman, *The San Francisco Labor Council Survey: Labor Plans for Health* (San Francisco: AF of San Francisco Labor Council, June 1952), catalogued collection, ILWU Library. Weinerman to Louis Goldblatt, 13 November 1953, and attached report, "Goals for a Health Center Program for the ILWU Welfare Fund." ILWU-PMA Welfare Fund secretary Goldie Krantz listed twenty-five union health centers in 1957, emphasizing medical society obstruction of the UMW and UAW programs. She singled

out the Chicago Building Service Employees plan and Teamster's Labor Health Institute in St. Louis as the only ones to provide complete medical services to employees and their families. Goldie Krantz to Union Trustees and International Officers (with note to "Harry" [Bridges]), 19 December 1957, History Files, Health and Welfare Proposals, ILWU Library.

43. Harry Becker to "Sid" Garfield, 30 November 1951, carton 78; Reuther to HJK, 28 January 1953, and 17 March 1953, carton 92; W. P. Reuther to HJK, 16 February 1954, carton 107, HJK Papers.

44. Garbarino, *Health Plans and Collective Bargaining*, 25, 216; report, Division of Labor Statistics and Research of the California Department of Industrial Relations and the Department of Preventive Medicine of the Stanford University School of Medicine, 1954, 13, catalogued collection, ILWU Library. UAW acting social security director James Brindle reported to the Wolverton Committee on Interstate and Foreign Commerce ("Stenographic Transcript of Hearings before the Committee on Interstate and Foreign Commerce—H.R., Washington, D.C., Monday, January 11, 1954," 7:87) that the "vast majority" of Ford and GM union members ultimately chose Kaiser when given dual choice. At the first election, only 15% at GM switched. But thereafter about 85% of all new workers chose Kaiser, and eventually an average of 55% had Kaiser coverage at the beginning of 1954. At Ford, he thought the percentage was "substantially higher." At Chrysler the dual choice agreement had been signed but not implemented at the time of the hearings, but Brindle said that the trend was increasingly to join Kaiser and that the union encouraged this since the Kaiser premium for the most comprehensive plan was below that of the most comprehensive Blue Cross plan. Copy of testimony in carton 108, HJK Papers.

45. Yedidia, Bancroft ROHO history, 49–55.

46. Poen, *Harry S. Truman*, 67–73; Donovan, *Conflict and Crisis*, 125–126, 212–218.

47. "Proposed Endorsement of President Truman's Health Message," n.d., c. 1945, carton 183; HJK to Mrs. Albert D. Lasker, 21 November 1945; Gerald Piel to Chad F. Calhoun, 8 January 1946, carton 33, HJK Papers. On the hearing, Poen, *Harry S. Truman*, 88–89.

48. Berkowitz, *America's Welfare State*, 161–162. Parran quoted in Stevens, *In Sickness and In Wealth*, 219–226. Stevens notes that by 1948 all states and territories except Nevada had submitted hospital surveys to the surgeon general. The 375 hospital regions covered 2,323 designated service areas, 104 of which were base hospital areas, at the apex of the research and education pyramids.

49. Fox argues that Hill-Burton was at odds with the regional hierarchy plan of the CCMC. It localized control of hospital policy on the pluralistic model of economic planning rather than the principle of universal access that characterized national health planning in the 1920s and 1930s. *Health Policies, Health Politics*, 130–131.

50. Stevens, *In Sickness and in Wealth*, 218–219.

51. Memo for File, 29 March 1945, carton 183, HJK Papers.

52. Ernest W. Saward interview by Sally Smith Hughes, 1985, Bancroft ROHO history, 57.

53. *California Board of Medical Examiners Directory 1947* (Sacramento) "Annual Report For 1946," 561. The case was reported in various stages of continuation and appeal through 1951, when a disposition was recorded on 5 May as follows: "License suspended for one year; provided that said

suspension shall be commuted to a period of one year during which period said suspension was stayed." In *California Board of Medical Examiners Directory, 1952*, "Annual Report For 1951," 698.

54. Unidentified clipping, "Chief to Take Row to Court," c. October 1947, carton 45, HJK Papers. Scott Fleming, *Kaiser-Permanente Medical Care Program History* (Kaiser Foundation Health Plan, 25 August 1983), 15.

55. Poen, *Harry S. Truman*, 170; Horace Hansen, Rolins, Davis, Lyons, and Hagen, to Dr. Sidney R. Garfield, 25 November 1947; Garfield to Hansen, 15 December 1947, carton 309, HJK Papers.

56. Horace Hansen, Rolins, Davis, Lyons, and Hagen, to Dr. Sidney R. Garfield, 25 November 1947; Garfield to Hansen, 15 December 1947, carton 309, HJK Papers.

57. ILWU *Dispatcher*, 5:22(31 October 1947), 2; "Memorandum for the file of conversation Farley with Yedidia of Permanente, 11 September 1947," ILWU Library, file: "Longshore Health Plans—Corres., Reports, Publicity, Misc. 1947–."

58. HJK to Frank A. Carvor, et al., 24 October 1947, carton 36, HJK Papers.

59. "Remarks made by Henry J. Kaiser before Doctors' Group, St. Francis Hotel," 9 June 1948, carton 103, HJK Papers.

60. Ibid.

61. Richard J. Walton, *Henry Wallace, Harry Truman, and the Cold War* (New York: Viking, 1976) for the pro-Wallace perspective on the election of 1948, and the liberal-progressive party split. "Year of Shocks" is the phrase of Eric F. Goldman, *The Crucial Decade—And After: America 1945–1960* (New York: Vintage, 1960). James M. Neil, M.D., Chairman of the California Medical Association Ethics Committee, to Judge, HJK, Garfield and Robert C. Elliott, 15 June 1949; E. E. Trefethen, Jr., to HJK, Garfield and Robert C. Elliott, 15 June 1949, saying decision would come in two months.

62. Dorothy M. Allen, M.D., and CMA to Harold H. Hitchcock, M.D., 10 November 1949, noting that charges are withdrawn, carton 45, HJK Papers. The court did finally rule that Garfield had violated the Medical Practices Act (99 C.A. 2d 219 [1950]). See Fleming, "Kaiser Permanente Program History," p. 15.

63. Fleming, "Kaiser Permanente Program History," 16; Morris F. Collen, M.D., interview by Sally Smith Hughes, 1986, Bancroft ROHO history, 42.

64. Collen, Bancroft ROHO history, 38–41.

65. HJK annotated drafts to Charles Wilson, Manley Fleischmann, and Oscar Ewing, 19 November 1951, carton 67; Wilson to HJK, 29 January 1952; draft letter HJK to Wilson, n.d., carton 77, HJK Papers.

66. Starr, *Social Transformation of American Medicine*, 359–360; Hanson W. Baldwin, "Medicine and Defense—An Analysis of How Physician Shortage is Affecting Morale of Armed Services," *New York Times*, 29 November 1955. Robert W. King, M.D., to Robert Elliott, 3 November 1955; telegram, Elliott to HJK, et al., 9 May and 8 October 1956; Clifford H. Keene to HJK, 26 November 1956, carton 124, HJK Papers.

67. Mimeo, notes on advisory committee, "Policy That No Doctor is 'Indispensable—for he might die,'" 19 February 1955, carton 89, HJK Papers.

68. Mimeo, "Military Installations and Defense Industries Personnel Require Services of Permanente Irreplaceable Key Doctors," n.d., c. late 1952,

carton 17, HJK Papers. The information in the following paragraph is also from this source.

69. HJK to Northern California Advisory Board, 28 August 1952; memo, Robert C. Elliott to Garfield, et al., 28 August 1952; HJK to Honorable Francis Whitehair, 6 October 1952; HJK to Dr. William L. Bender, 14 October 1952; HJK to Vice Admiral L. T. DuBose, 26 November 1952; DuBose to HJK, 2 December 1952; Frances P. Whitehair to HJK, 20 December 1952; Charles Thomas to HJK, 31 March 1953; HJK to Admiral B. F. Rodgers, 20 May 1953; Chief of Naval Personnel to Pellegrin, 6 July 1953, carton 89, HJK Papers.

70. "Confidential" memo, 18 March 1955 on HJK telephone conversation with Hershey, carton 116; Garfield to Harold Morse, M.D., Chairman Alameda-Contra Costa Medical Advisory Committee, 5 February 1954; Col. R. L. Black to Garfield, 14 January 1955, carton 77; Kaiser to Local Board No. 49 (in Garfield's behalf), 13 April 1954, carton 104; mimeo, "Our Meeting With President's National Selective Service Appeal Board," 6 December 1955; carton 116, HJK Papers.

71. Elliott report to HJK, 14 September 1956; Elliott to Dr. Robert King, et al., 1 February 1956, carton 124, HJK Papers.

72. Winnie C. Ware, Local Board No. 30, to HJK, 15 February 1957, carton 124; Frederick A. Pellegrin to "Mr. Kaiser," 13 September 1956, carton 247, HJK Papers.

73. Eisenhower quoted in Poen, *Harry S. Truman*, 207. Teletype to HJK, 10 March 1953; memo, Chad F. Calhoun to HJK, 18 March 1953, carton 88, HJK Papers. Davis, *Medical Care for Tomorrow*, 293.

74. Memo, Chad F. Calhoun to HJK, 18 March 1953, carton 88, HJK Papers.

75. Bess Furman, "Mrs. Hobby to Set Health Policies; She Favors Voluntary Programs," *New York Times*, 10 May 1953; "Health Services Faces A 'Staggering' Job," *New York Times*, 10 May 1953, 1.

76. Stephen E. Ambrose, *Eisenhower: The President* (New York: Simon & Schuster, 1984), 64; William E. Leuchtenburg, *A Troubled Feast: American Society Since 1945* (Boston: Little, Brown, 1979), 9, 45–55, 65, 75.

77. Mimeo, "Unbudgeted Expenditures May Result in Kaiser Foundation Cash Balance Deficit for 1954," 31 December 1953, carton 90, HJK Papers; memo, Chad F. Calhoun to Governor Sherman Adams, 27 January 1953, Official File, Box 598, Folder Health-1, White House Central Files, Dwight D. Eisenhower Library, Abilene, Kansas. Also, mimeo, "Opportunities for Doctors and Position of Doctors on H.R. 7700," n.a., n.d., carton 108; mimeo of speech, 18 November 1953, "Medical Group Facilities and Hospital Mortgage Loan Insurance Act—To Establish Mortgage Loan Insurance Enabling Doctors through Investment of Private Capital To Build and Equip Hospitals and Other Medical Facilities and To Extend Voluntary, Pre-Payment Health Plans Providing Comprehensive Medical and Hospital Care," carton 88, HJK Papers.

78. Mimeo of Hobby remarks, Calhoun to HJK, 2 January 1953, carton 88, HJK Papers.

79. HJK to Oveta Culp Hobby, 25 August 1953, carton 89; mimeo, "A Nation-Wide Medical Center Plan—First Draft of HJK Remarks to Press Conference for Los Angeles Hospital Opening," 19 May 1953, carton 91; Robert C. Elliott to HJK re. Cruikshank wire, 29 September 1953, carton 93, HJK Papers.

80. Mimeo draft, "Hospital Loan Insurance Bill," 12 November 1953, carton 89; Elliott to HJK, 14 November 1953; mimeo, "Medical Group Facilities and Hospital Mortgage Loan Insurance Act," 18 November 1953, carton 88; Elliott to Calhoun, 30 November 1953, carton 93; mimeo, "Opportunities For Doctors and Position of Doctors on H.R. 7700," n.d., carton 108, HJK Papers.

81. Calhoun to HJK, 11 January 1954; Walton Cloke, news release, 11 January 1954; memo, Cloke to HJK, 12 January 1954; *Kaiser Washington Report* 4:1(15 January 1954), carton 107, HJK Papers; "Henry Kaiser Proposes New Hospital Plan," Washington *Times-Herald*, 12 January 1954. Mimeo, "From the President's State of the Union Address," 7 January 1954, carton 107; teletype, Calhoun to HJK, 7 January 1954, carton 103, HJK Papers.

82. Memo report of meeting, Calhoun to HJK, 12 January 1954, carton 107; teletype, Calhoun to HJK, 18 January 1954, and Calhoun to HJK, 28 January 1954, carton 103, HJK Papers; Ray Bruner, "Mrs. Hobby Sights Doom of Compulsory Insurance," *Toledo Blade*, 12 March 1954.

83. HJK to Walter Reuther, 9 February 1954; Reuther to HJK, 16 February 1954; Walter T. Phair to Arthur Weissman re. Nelson H. Cruikshank testimony before Wolverton Committee, 31 March 1954, carton 107, HJK Papers. "Reinsurance Plan Would Not Solve Nation's Health Problem, AFL says," *Journal of Commerce*, 2 April 1954, carton 108, HJK Papers.

84. Memo, Elliott to HJK, 15 April 1954; teletype, Calhoun to HJK, 16 April 1954, carton 107, HJK Papers. On the Bank of America, Wally Phair to HJK, 5 May 1954; teletype, Calhoun to HJK, 7 May 1954; memo, E. E. Trefethen to HJK, 11 May 1954; Phair to HJK, 14 May 1954, carton 107, HJK Papers.

85. "The New Economics of Medical Care," Henry J. Kaiser Address to the National Press Club, Washington, D.C., 26 May 1954, carton 108, HJK Papers.

86. Mimeo, "Henry J. Kaiser Statement—Opposition to Group Practice Prepayment Plans Based on Fear of Free Competition," April 1954; news release, 30 April 1954, carton 107, HJK Papers; "Kaiser Backs Group Practice by Physicians," *Corpus Christie Times*, 30 April 1954; "Personalities," *Dayton News*, 30 April 1954; "Kaiser Urges More Prepaid Health Plans," *Washington Post, Times-Herald*, 1 May 1954; "Kaiser Gives Backing to Ike Health Plan," San Francisco *Chronicle*, 1 May 1954.

87. Calhoun to Trefethen, 3 May 1954; teletype, Calhoun to HJK, 28 June 1954; memo, Calhoun to HJK, 6 July 1954; teletype, Calhoun to HJK, 13 July 1954, carton 107, HJK Papers.

88. Mimeo, "Bills to Establish Government FHA Type Insurance of Loans for Medical Facilities are Pending in Congress in the following forms," 31 January 1955; "AMA Statement on Health Message," *Congressional Record*, 25 February 1955, excerpt; H. Walton Cloke to Calhoun, 7 February 1954, carton 116, HJK Papers; "Text of the President's Health Message to Congress," *New York Times*, 1 February 1955; Russell Baker, "Health Insurance Poses a National Problem," *New York Times*, 6 February 1955; Cabell Phillips, "President's Program Enters Critical Phase—G.O.P. Election Perils Loom Unless Congress Speeds Legislature Pace," *New York Times*, 30 May 1954.

89. Memo, Calhoun to HJK, 25 June 1954; Calhoun to HJK, 24 August 1954, carton 107, HJK Papers.

90. HJK to Elliott, 8 January 1955; Elliott to HJK, 2 March 1955, carton 116; HJK to Calhoun, 17 January 1955, carton 117, HJK Papers.
91. Personal memo, HJK to Calhoun, 17 October 1955; Calhoun to HJK, 26 January 1956; Scott Fleming to Directors, KFHP, 25 March 1957; Fleming to Phair, 19 May 1958; Fleming to Phair, 14 May 1958, carton 268, HJK Papers.

4   Henry Kaiser Takes Charge

1. Stub Stollery to Trefethen, 30 October 1952; A. B. Ordway to Edgar Kaiser, Trefethen and Kaiser attorneys, 7 November 1952, carton 78, HJK Papers. Memo, Edgar Kaiser, et al., from A. B. Ordway, 6 November 1952, carton 92:20, EFK Papers. Scott Fleming describes this action as "unilateral" in "Kaiser-Permanente Program History," 23–24. Raymond M. Kay also holds this view. See Kay interview by Foster and Kay, *Historical Review*, 79–80.
2. Foster, *Henry J. Kaiser*, 133–135, 126; Hall, *Cities of Tomorrow*, quotation from Mumford (1925), 148–152, also 294–295. Connection with regionalism in medical care is drawn from Fox, *Health Policies, Health Politics*, 19.
3. Hall, *Cities of Tomorrow*, quote from Mumford (1925), 148–152.
4. Stub Stollery to Trefethen, 30 October 1952; A. B. Ordway to Edgar Kaiser, Trefethen and Kaiser attorneys, 7 November 1952, carton 78, HJK Papers. Memo, Edgar Kaiser, et al., from A. B. Ordway, 6 November 1952, carton 92:20, EFK Papers.
5. Berkowitz, *America's Welfare State*, 163.
6. Harvard refused $1.5 million in 1913, when the GEB tied it to fulfillment of recommendations in the Flexner Report that full-time replace the traditional part-time faculty system. On Flexner's influence in the Bay Area, see William G. Rothstein, *American Medical Schools and the Practice of Medicine—A History* (New York: Oxford University Press, 1987), 162–168; Scott, *San Francisco Bay Area*, 53–55.
7. Rickey Hendricks, "The History of UCSF to 1950," August 1990 (work in progress); Lloyd Smith address on the history of UCSF, 10 November 1989, San Francisco.
8. Paul Scholten, "The Founding of UCSF," 20–21, and Malcolm S. M. Watts, "The Volunteer Teaching Faculty at UCSF," *San Francisco Medicine* 62:9 (September 1989), 29.
9. Scott, *San Francisco Bay Area*, 82–83; Fleming interview by author.
10. Kay, *Historical Review*, 19.
11. Clyde F. Diddle, memo, "Formal Patient Complaints," to M. F. Collen, M.D., 13 November 1952; HJK memo to Garfield, 18 November 1952, carton 77, HJK Papers.
12. Memo, Goldie Krantz to Union Trustees and International Officers, 19 December 1957, marked "Harry" [Bridges], History Files, Health and Welfare Proposals, ILWU Library.
13. Fred Grimm, "Coal Miners Struggle for Union's Future," *Miami Herald*, 8 July 1989, 1, 6A; Robert H. Zeiger, *John L. Lewis—Labor Leader* (Boston: Twayne, 1988), 150–179; Boone, *Medical Survey of the Bituminous-Coal Industry*, 115–119; typescript, "Medical-Hospital Problems in the Bituminous Coal Mine Areas of Kentucky, Tennessee, and West Virginia," submitted 16 June 1952, to the AMA Committee on Medical Care for Industrial

Workers by an investigative team of physicians, Series 3, Executive Medical Officer Subject Files [hereafter Series 3], Council on Medical Service, UMW Survey Report, box 7 of 52, file folder [hereafter ff.] 4, UMWA Archives.

14.   "The Gate of Bright Hope," (*Reader's Digest?*), May 1948, carton 309; memo on Kabat-Kaiser history, n.d.; Garfield to W. R. Price, Jr., telephone dictation from unidentified caller to *Times Herald*, Washington, D.C., 30 June 1946; "Helping Them to Walk Again," 1952 exhibit for UMW convention, Cincinnati, carton 309, HJK Papers.

15.   Table, Permanente Hospitals and Kabat-Kaiser Institute, "Analysis of Changes to United Mine Workers of America compared with Value of Services Rendered, January through September 1952," Series III: Executive Medical Officer—Subject Files—Permanente Foundation Hospital Policy, Box 24, File Folder 13, UMWA Archives; Warren F. Draper, M.D., to Vallejo patient, 15 December 1949, ibid., Box 14, File Folder 2.

16.   Garfield interview by Stein, 28. Clifford Keene, interview conducted in 1985 by Sally Smith Hughes, Bancroft ROHO history, 1986, 51–52.

17.   Elliott to HJK, E. E. Trefethen, Jr., Garfield, 31 January 1950; Elliott to same and Edgar Kaiser, 6 February 1950, carton 56; memo, "Plan to Unite AMA and Permanente," 7 July 1951, carton 5, HJK Papers.

18.   Notes, "Talk with Dr. Cline, 5 July 1951," hand addressed to Mr. H. J. Kaiser and signed by Paul de Kruif; memo Trefethen to HJK, Garfield, 23 July 1951; memo, de Kruif to HJK, Jr., "Conference at Wake Robin, July 20–22 with Drs. Elmer L. Henderson and George F. Lull," 23 July 1951, carton 67, HJK Papers.

19.   Collen, Bancroft ROHO history, 17.

20.   Mimeo, "Brief Resume of Dinner Meeting Held by Dr. Chandler on Tuesday Night," 31 July 1951; Trefethen to Chandler, 4 August 1951, carton 77, HJK Papers.

21.   Fleming conversation with author, 16 March 1989.

22.   Ibid.

23.   *California Board of Medical Examiners Directory*, 1947–50; mimeo, Trefethen to Dr. Richard Bullis, 24 January 1952, carton 77, HJK Papers.

24.   Memo, Garfield to Kaiser, 14 March 1952; memo, Trefethen to Board of Trustees, Henry J. Kaiser Family Foundation, 7 November 1952, carton 77, HJK Papers.

25.   Not until the late 1980s would Kaiser Permanente establish working ties with Stanford University, and then with the business school rather than the school of medicine. Fleming conversation with author, 16 March 1989.

26.   For changes in the nursing profession and more stringent licensing requirements see Barbara Melosh, *'The Physician's Hand': Work Culture and Conflict in American Nursing* (Philadelphia: Temple University Press, 1982). The Kaiser organization found other ways to contribute to education. The foundation, medical group, and health plan made a study of how the Women's Medical College [of Philadelphia] could institute a program on the Kaiser Permanente group practice model. The Kaiser Family Foundation set up a premedical scholarship at St. Mary's College, and a $20,000 nursing and medical education scholarship at the Punahou School near a new Kaiser residence at Oahu, Hawaii. A $20,000 donation also was made to the Cordell Hull Foundation for U.S. medical students. See memo, Eaton M. MacKay, M.D., to HJK, 27 January 1953, carton 91; memo, Collen to HJK, 12 June 1953, carton 89; mimeo, "Opportunities Presented by a Medical

Center Health Plan for Women's Medical College and Hospital," n.d., c. 1953, carton 93; news release, 21 January 1954; C. Dudley Pratt to HJK, 31 December 1954, carton 106, HJK Papers.

27.   Garfield interview by Stein; memo, Walter T. Phair to HJK, n.d., rejecting Nursing Education Act of 1953, carton 88, HJK Papers.

28.   In 1900 24% of all deaths were categorized as attributable to chronic disease, 76% to infectious diseases; the percentages were 34% and 66% in 1920; 68% and 32% in 1945. President's Commission on the Health Needs of the Nation, *Building America's Health*, vol. 3 (Washington, D.C., 1951), 30. Quoted in Stevens, *In Sickness and In Wealth*, 203, 397n13.

29.   Collen, Bancroft ROHO history, 29–30.

30.   Milton Silverman, "The Arginase Story—Facts Show Drug Won't Help Cancer," San Francisco *Chronicle*, 25 February 1952; Ved Vrat to HJK; HJK, Jr., to Garfield and MacKay, 30 April 1952; Vrat to Mr. and Mrs. Henry J. Kaiser, 23 August 1952; Eaton M. MacKay, M.D., to Garfield, 22 June 1952, carton 78, HJK Papers.

31.   Jac Lessman to HJK, 16 October 1952; Lessman to HJK, 21 October 1952; Kaiser to Lessman, 17 October 1952; MacKay to HJK, 12 November 1952; memo, Kaiser to Garfield, 14 November 1952; A. L. Baritell, M.D., to HJK, 3 December 1952; Lessman to HJK, 11 December 1952; Lessman to Garfield, 25 November 1952; Lessman to HJK, 25 November 1951; HJK to Lessman, 26 November 1952, carton 78, HJK Papers.

32.   Yedidia, Bancroft ROHO history, 68–69.

33.   The most frequent diagnoses (5%) were for vision, blood pressure, and electrocardiogram tests; 2% had hearing problems. Less than 1% had problems revealed by chest x-rays, serologic tests for syphilis, blood and urine sugar, and urine albumen. A striking 20% were overweight, increasing the incidence of many of the other ailments. See E. Richard Weinerman, Lester Breslow, Nedra B. Belloc, Anne Waybur, and Benno K. Milmore, "Multiphasic Screening of Longshoremen with Organized Medical Follow-up," *American Journal of Public Health*, 42:12(December 1952), 1552–1567.

34.   Memo, HJK to Bullis, 15 September 1952; memo, HJK to Garfield, 22 September 1952; memo, Bullis to HJK, 22 September 1952, carton 77, HJK Papers.

35.   Kay, *Historical Review*, 80.

36.   Kay interview by Foster.

37.   Cutting, "Kaiser-Permanente Program History," 20–21, 47.

38.   AMA, *Organized Payments of Medical Services*, 12–14.

39.   Fleming interview by Foster, 10 January 1984; Fleming interview by author, 16 March 1989.

40.   Thomas K. McCarthy to HJK, 10 December 1952, with "Description of Method of Operation of the Permanente Health Plan," and "Comments on Methods of Operation . . .," carton 77, HJK Papers; "Kaiser Foundation Medical Centers and Health Plan Prepared for the Women's Medical College, Kaiser Conference," 12 January 1953, Series 3, UMWA Archives. Average U.S. physician salary was estimated at $13,432 in 1951 according to Rothstein, *American Medical Schools*, 190, table 9.1.

41.   "County Medical Societies' Refusal for Memberships to Doctors Serving Kaiser Foundation Health Plan Members"; "Doctors Blocked from Specialist Boards Because They Are Refused County Medical Membership"; "Warnings to Our Doctors or Those Interested in Group Practice," carton 89, HJK Papers.

42. "Doctors Blocked from Specialist Boards."

43. Ibid.; "County Medical Societies' Refusal for Memberships to Doctors Serving Kaiser Foundation Health Plan Members." Paul de Kruif, "Talk with Dr. Cline," 5 July 1951, carton 67, HJK Papers.

44. De Kruif, "Talk with Dr. Cline."

45. Collen, Bancroft ROHO history, 52–53; "Bay Area Proposal."

46. Collen, Bancroft ROHO history, 52–53.

47. An overview is Robert J. Donovan, *Tumultuous Years: The Presidency of Harry S Truman, 1949–1953* (New York: Norton, 1982), 26–27, 162–175.

48. E. R. Weinerman to Garfield, n.d., c. 1951, box 29:26, E. R. Weinerman Papers, Sterling Library, Yale University [hereafter Weinerman Papers].

49. Ernest Besig, Director Northern California ACLU, to HJK, Garfield, and Trustees, 8 October 1951, carton 67, HJK Papers.

50. Quote from John G. Smillie, *Can Physicians Manage the Quality and Costs of Health Care?* (New York: McGraw-Hill, 1991), 118; "California Institute of Physical Medicine and Rehabilitation, Vallejo, California," 15 January 1954, carton 103:23, EFK Papers.

51. Weinerman notes, "Discussion of 11 September 1951," box 29:86, Weinerman Papers. Weinerman, *San Francisco Labor Council Survey.* Leslie A. Falk, "E. Richard Weinerman, M.D., M.P.H. (July 17, 1917–February 21, 1970)," *Yale Journal of Biology and Medicine* 44 (August, 1971). Arthur J. Viseltear remarks to author, 26 April 1989.

52. Collen, Bancroft ROHO history, 54–55; Ephraim Kahn, Bancroft ROHO history, taped interview, not transcribed, conducted in 1985 by Ora Huth; Alice D. Friedman, M.D., interview conducted in 1986 by Sally Smith Hughes, 1987, Bancroft ROHO history, 29.

53. Gladys Nitzberg to HJK, 9 September 1951, carton 67, HJK Papers.

54. Mimeo, untitled, unsigned, 21 February 1952, probably a report by a Permanente "plant" in the meeting, carton 77, HJK Papers. Handwritten notes, restricted, n.t., n.d., "Northern California District Council Files, Permanente Subcommittee, 1951–53," ILWU Library.

55. Handwritten notes, restricted, n.t., n.d., "Northern California District Council Files, Permanente Subcommittee, 1951–53," ILWU Library. (Names not already public knowledge have been removed from this file.)

56. Collen, Bancroft ROHO history, 54–55.

57. Flyer received by Ship Clerks Association, Local 34, c. 2 February 1952, "Northern California District Council Files, Permanente Subcommittee," ILWU Library.

58. Mimeo, untitled, unsigned, 21 February 1952, probably a report by a Permanente "plant" in the meeting, carton 77, HJK Papers.

59. Documents in "Northern California District Council Files, Permanente Subcommittee," ILWU Library.

60. Scott Fleming interview by Mark S. Foster, 10 January 1984.

61. For this breakdown see E. Richard Weinerman typescript, "The Permanente Medical Plan," 27 July 1951, box 29: 85, Weinerman Papers.

62. Saward, Bancroft ROHO history, 86.

63. Cutting, Bancroft ROHO history, 33.

64. Report, Weinerman to Garfield, "General Critical Observations of the Permanente Health Plan," n.d., c. 1951, marked "Confidential—Not For Public Release," and attachment, box 29:86, Weinerman Papers.

65. Ibid.

66. Ibid.

67. Raymond Kay to Sidney R. Garfield, 10 September 1951, box 29:86, Weinerman Papers.

68. E. Richard Weinerman, draft of "Discussion of 11 September 1951," box 29:86, Weinerman Papers. Subsequent references to this discussion and to rebutting remarks are cited in the text as Weinerman.

69. Garbarino, *Health Plans and Collective Bargaining*, 151–157. Weinerman published *Labor Plans For Health* in 1952.

5 Medical Practice Embattled

1. Estimates from table, "Total Health Plan Membership January 1953–June 1955," carton 117, HJK Papers; table, "Kaiser Foundation Health Plan Membership," 1950–63, carton 247, HJK Papers; "Kaiser Foundation Health Plan, Southern California Division, Utilization of Facilities by Membership through Retail Clerks, Culinary Group and Longshore Groups," by month, July 1953 to December 1955; "Kaiser Foundation Health Plan, Southern California Division, Utilization Statistics Per Member per Year," 1953–55, carton 132:21, EFK Papers. "Attachment to BLS 2290, U.S. Dept. of Labor"; "Summary of ILWU–PMA Welfare Plan," March 1953, History Files, ILWU Library. Garbarino, *Health Plans and Collective Bargaining*, 27; DeSilva, "Need A Doctor?"

2. Table, "Health Plan Membership for Selected Years," carton 339; mimeo, "Essential Key Physician Executives," summary statement by Permanente Medical Groups, Kaiser Foundation Health Plan, 6 December 1955, carton 309, HJK Papers. Fleming, "Kaiser-Permanente Program History," 7, 10; Somers, *Kaiser-Permanente Medical Care Program*, 199 (table 5).

3. Trauner, "From Benevolence to Negotiation," 142–166.

4. Editorial, *California Medicine*, 78 (January 1953).

5. Kay, *Historical Review*, 132.

6. Paul D. Foster, "Outlooks for Medicine," *Bulletin* of the Los Angeles County Medical Association [hereafter LACMA *Bulletin*], 5 Mar. 1953, 231, 256–259.

7. "A.M.A. Declares War—The Challenge Is Accepted," n.a., 26 March 1953, carton 92, HJK Papers.

8. Chad C. Calhoun to HJK, Trefethen, and Garfield, 27 March 1953, ibid.

9. Foster, "Proposed Resolution For the Consideration of the Council," 20 April 1953, carton 91, HJK Papers.

10. *JAMA* 155 (31 July 1954), 1249. Apparently deferred by Commission on Medical Care Plans, Leonard W. Larson, M.D., chair, in December 1954.

11. William G. Riley to Paul J. Steil, 14 May 1953, carton 91, HJK Papers.

12. Collen, Bancroft ROHO history, 81–82.

13. "Our President Says," LACMA *Bulletin*, 21 May 1953, 501.

14. McCarthy to Elliott, et al., 6, 7 August 1953, carton 92, HJK Papers.

15. *Group Health Cooperative of Puget Sound v. King County Medical Society*, 39 Wash. 2d 586, 237 P.2d 137(1951). Hyde and Wolff, "American Medical Association," 992. "Summary of ILWU–PMA Welfare Plan, 1953," Health Plans—Brochures, 1953–69; "Attachment to BLS 2290, U.S. Department

of Labor," U.S. Labor Dept. Questionnaires, 1953–58, History Files, ILWU Library.

16. *San Diego Union*, 8 March 1952; "Comment—Medical Service Plans in California," *California Law Review*, 43 (1953), 675–686; "Medical Martyr or Malpractitioner?" *Fortnight*, September 1956, 45.

17. McCarthy to Garfield, 12 October 1953, carton 92, HJK Papers; George E. Link to Trustees, 15 December 1954, carton 132:21, EFK Papers. Burnham, "American Medicine's Golden Age," 1474–79.

18. Editorial, "Kaiser Deserves Hospital Lease," Long Beach *Labor News*, 10 April 1953.

19. "Doctors Plan Leaflet Distributed to Voting Steelworkers," 3 September 1953; Local 1440, "Insurance Committee," carton 92, HJK Papers; Neil Dickson, "Whoop-Te-Do Ends; Steelworkers Flock to Vote for Medical Scheme," Pittsburg *Post-Dispatch*, 4 September 1953.

20. "Doctors Outline Insurance Plan"; George Duschece, "CPS in Southland Expands Coverage," *San Francisco News*, 14 December 1953; "Doctors OK Congress Red-Hunt in Schools," Milton Silverman, "CMA Told Kaiser Has Lost at Douglas Plant," and "Kaiser Hails the CMA Victory," San Francisco *Chronicle*, 15 December 1953.

21. "Doctors, Union Fund Sign Up," *Business Week*, 30 July 1955, 78. The San Joaquin County Medical Society–CPS plan started in 1955 for a group of 521 longshoremen. The union pressured local doctors to start the plan by threatening to start a Kaiser plan. "Attachment to BLS 2290, U.S. Dept. of Labor," ILWU Library. Somers, *Kaiser-Permanente Medical Care Program*, 178.

22. Kenneth P. Andrews, "How They're Fighting the Kaiser Plan," *Medical Economics* 31 (September 1954), 122–130. "Welfare Fund Offers Plan in LA Harbor," ILWU *Dispatcher* 14 (25 May 1956), 2; "San Pedro ILWU Hails New Port Hospital," ibid. (7 December 1956), 5.

23. Jack Howard, "AFL Warns Doctors to Re-examine Policies," San Francisco *Chronicle*, 22 March 1952. "Sneak Attack Made on Kaiser Plan," Long Beach *Labor News*, 24 April 1953. Paul Ditzel, "Labor Unions Irate as Health Centers Hit," Los Angeles *Daily News*, n.d., note that copies made 10 October 1953, carton 92, HJK Papers. "Medical Relations, re: report by John Hutchinsons," 1 April 1954, carton 105, HJK Papers.

24. *Look* articles 5 September 1952, 15 December 1953. Kaiser editorial courtesies by the press, "Kaiser Health Plan Draft of *Look* Article as corrected by us," 10 April 1952; Lester Velie, "Supermarket Medicine," *Saturday Evening Post*, 20 June 1953, 20–50; "Chet Huntley—American Broadcasting Co.," 10 September 1952, carton 78, HJK Papers. See also Norman Thomas, "Any Truce Preferable to Continued Conflict," *Oakland Tribune*, 11 June 1953; special series by Hale Champion, San Francisco *Chronicle*, 14, 15, 16 February 1954.

25. Norman Vincent Peale to HJK, 29 November 1949, carton 43, HJK Papers; mimeo, "Education Work on Behalf of the Kaiser Health Work," n.a., n.d., but c. 1951, carton 67, HJK Papers. Peale quoted in Richard Weiss, *The Myth of Success: From Alger Hiss to Norman Vincent Peale* (New York: Basic Books, 1969), 223.

26. Velie, "Supermarket Medicine," 20; mimeo, "Possible Questions on Saturday Evening Post Articles," n.d.; mimeo, "A Nation-Wide Medical Center Plan—First Draft of HJK Remarks to Press Conference for Los Angeles Hospital Opening," 19 May 1953, carton 91, HJK Papers.

27. Friedman, Bancroft ROHO history, 21–25.

28. Ora Thelen Gillingham to "Mr. Kaiser," 24 July 1951; Stephen Charter to Kaiser, 8 September 1951.

29. Sara Lee Silberman, "Pioneering in Family-Centered Maternity and Infant Care: Edith B. Jackson and the Yale Rooming-In Research Project," *Bulletin of the History of Medicine* 64 (1990), 262–287 (quotes and references, 283–287). L. Emmett Holt, *The Care and Feeding of Children: A Catechism for the Use of Mothers and Children's Nurses*, 10th ed., rev and enl. (New York: D. Appleton, 1920), 192–193. Benjamin Spock, *The Common Sense Book of Baby and Child Care* (New York: Duell, Sloan and Pearce, 1946). Judith Walzer Leavitt, *Brought to Bed; Child-Bearing in America, 1750–1950* (New York: Oxford University Press, 1986), 171.

30. Press releases, 12 June 1951 and April 16, 1952, featuring "Private Nursing Plan," carton 67, HJK Papers.

31. Typescript, "Kaiser Health Plan Draft of *Look* Article as corrected by us," 10 April 1952, carton 78, HJK Papers. The *Look* articles appeared on 5 September 1952, and 15 December 1953.

32. Betty de Losada, History Files, Warehouse Welfare, ILWU Library; E. Richard Weinerman, San Francisco Labor Council Survey, *Labor Plans For Health* (San Francisco, June 1952), 11; "Labor-Management Health Plans Which Include Kaiser Foundation Health Plan in Dual Choice Program," c. 1956, carton 117, HJK Papers; Garbarino, *Health Plans and Collective Bargaining*, 25, 216.

33. HJK to Governor Earl Warren, 10 February 1949; Walter D. Fuller to HJK, 6 November, 20, 4 December 1951; Jack Cracknell to Permanente, 7 November 1951, carton 67, HJK Papers. Mea Heckrotte to HJK, 17 August 1949, carton 45, HJK Papers.

34. Report, "Kaiser Foundation Psychiatric Clinic," September 1954, carton 105, HJK Papers; Nygren and Childs, *Federal Employees' Health Benefits Program*, 2. Kaiser's reluctance in this field of health care is notable in light of the considerable recognition by the medical profession and government of postwar mental health needs.

35. Ben Pearse, "What Has John L. Lewis Done with His $400,000,000?" *Saturday Evening Post*, 30 August 1952, 26.

36. Report from Warren F. Draper to the Council on Medical Service, American Medical Association, 11 February 1952, Series II: Executive Medical Officer Subject Files—AMA Council on Medical Service 1949–1952, Box 16, File Folder 4, UMWA Archives. Todd Inch, "Report on Key Management and Doctor Personnel for Miner's Hospital Program," n.d., c. 1951; "Kaiser Permanente Hospitals for United Mine Workers Welfare Fund," notebook marked "confidential draft" and "Organization Planning to Extend Kaiser-Permanente Work," carton 67, HJK Papers.

37. Inch, "Report on Key Management"; "Kaiser Permanente Hospitals for United Mine Workers Welfare Fund," notebook marked "confidential draft" and "Organization Planning to Extend Kaiser-Permanente Work," carton 67, HJK Papers; mimeo, "Notes on Conference with Dr. Sidney Garfield at Washington Office May 4, 1951," Series 3, Permanente Foundation Hospital, Dental, box 14, ff. 9, UMWA Archives.

38. W. A. Sawyer, M.D., Medical Consultant, Eastman Kodak Company and Chairman of the AMA Committee on Medical Care for Industrial Workers, to Warren F. Draper, 18 June 1952; preliminary draft, "Medical-Hospital Problems in the Bituminous Coal Mine Areas of Kentucky,

Tennessee, and West Virginia," submitted 16 June 1952 to the AMA Committee on Medical Care for Industrial Workers, by the investigating team (marked "Confidential—not to be released in part or full in any manner"), Series 3, AMA Committee on Medical Care for Industrial Workers, 1949–1952, box 16 of 52, ff. 2, UMWA Archives. Final recommendations of the survey team reported in *JAMA* 151, 407–412, 848–849.

39. "Henry J. Kaiser comments on the UMW proposal for Permanente Hospital Services, 13 July 1951, made in discussion with Dr. Sidney R. Garfield, Dr. Cecil Cutting, and Henry J. Kaiser, Jr., carton 67, HJK Papers.

40. Zeiger, *John L. Lewis*, 160–161; "Henry J. Kaiser comments," carton 67, HJK Papers.

41. Garfield interview by Foster.

42. HJK remarks, "John L. Lewis, United Mine Workers Medical Insurance Plan," carton 67, HJK Papers.

43. Memo, Goldie Krantz to Union Trustees and International Officers, 19 December 1957, History Files, Health and Welfare Proposals, ILWU Library; memo and form letter, Warren F. Draper, M.D., to Area Medical Administrators, Re: Recruitment of Physicians for Group Practice Clinics, 9 December 1964, Series 3, box 14 of 52, ff. Miscellaneous 1952–1964, UMWA Archives.

44. HJK remarks, "John L. Lewis, United Mine Workers Medical Insurance Plan," carton 67, HJK Papers.

45. Memo, H. Walton Cloke, Coordinator Public Relations, Kaiser Companies, to HJK, 27 May 1954, carton 108, HJK Papers. Josephine Roche to Doctor Draper, 2 June 1954; handwritten note, Draper to Morrison, 10 June 1954, Series 3, Hospital and Medical Care Agencies, Kabat-Kaiser Institute, California, Publicity, Publications, box 6, ff. 1, UMWA Archives.

46. John L. Lewis to Henry J. Kaiser, 2 June 1954, Series 3, Hospitals and Medical Care Agencies, Kabat-Kaiser Institute, California, Publicity, Publications, box 6 of 6, ff. 1, UMWA Archives.

47. Interoffice memos, Doctor Draper to Miss Roche, 2 June 1954; HJK to John L. Lewis, 10 June 1954; see also correspondence between Garfield and Draper: Draper to Garfield, 2 June 1954; Garfield to Draper, 21 June 1954, ibid.

48. Memo, Dr. Draper to Miss Roche, 26 June 1951; Draper to Roche, 18 July 1951; Garfield to Draper, 18 July 1951; Draper to Garfield, 18 July 1951, ibid., Permanente Foundation Hospitals, Sidney R. Garfield, MD, Project, box 14 of 52, ff. 15.

49. Davis, *Medical Care For Tomorrow*, 234–235. Subsequently, the union trustees formed the Miners Memorial Hospital Association of ten hospitals in Kentucky, Virginia, and West Virginia, but then transferred them to the incorporated Appalachian Regional Hospitals in 1964. Memo, Warren F. Draper, M.D., to Area Medical Administrators, Re: Recruitment of Physicians for Group Practice Clinics, 9 December 1964; form letter, Draper to interested physicians, n.d., Series 3, box 14 of 52, ff. Miscellaneous, 1952–1964, UMWA Archives.

50. Zeiger, *John L. Lewis*, 172–173.

51. The AMA warning was published in 1959, but the commission study that generated it began in 1954, under Larson. It appeared in *JAMA*, special edition, part 1, 17 January 1959, 37–38. The cases were *AMA v. U.S.*, 317 U.S.519 (1943); *U.S. v. Oregon State Medical Society*, 39 Wash2d 586, 237 P.2d

737(1951) reh.den(1952); *Complete Service Bureau v. San Diego County Medical Society*, 43 Cal.2d 201, 272 P.2d 497(1954).

52. Elliott quoting Garfield in memo to HJK, 24 September 1954, carton 103, HJK Papers; Saward to the author, September 1987.

53. Clifford H. Keene, M.D., to George F. Lull, M.D. [Secretary AMA Judicial Council], 31 March 1954, carton 105, HJK Papers.

54. These social contexts are explored in Rosenberg, *The Care of Strangers*, 5, 47–51.

55. Memos, HJK to Trefethen, and HJK to Garfield, 19 October 1953, carton 19, HJK Papers.

56. Viseltear, "The Definition of Public Health," in Numbers, *Compulsory Health Insurance*, 27, 29, 41, 44–46.

57. Draft of E. Richard Weinerman, M.D., speech to the Northern Permanente doctors, 11 September 1951, box 29:86, Weinerman Papers.

58. Cutting interview by Foster; Fleming interview by Foster.

59. Thomas K. McCarthy to Henry J. Kaiser, 10 December 1952, with mimeos, "Description of Method of Operation of the Permanente Health Plan," and "Comments on Methods of Operation . . .," carton 77, HJK Papers. Average U.S. physician salary was estimated at $13,432 in 1951. Rothstein, *American Medical Schools*, 190 (table 9.1).

60. Mimeo, "Remarks of Henry J. Kaiser to Be Given at Walnut Creek, 15 May 1953," carton 93, HJK Papers.

61. Garfield interview by Stein, 29.

62. Garfield interview by Foster.

63. Trefethen, Bancroft ROHO history, 34; Garfield interview by Stein, 29.

64. HJK to John F. Tomayko, Contract Department, United Steelworkers, 29 July 1953; HJK to "Mr. Fairless," 2 February 1954, carton 106, HJK Papers.

65. Garfield interview by Stein, 29–30; mimeo, "Unbudgeted Expenditures May Result in Kaiser Foundation Cash Balance Deficit for 1954," 31 December 1953, carton 90, HJK Papers.

66. Mimeo, c. 12 December 1953, "Unbudgeted Expenditures May Result in Kaiser Foundation Cash Balance Deficit For 1954," carton 90; memos, HJK to J. F. Reise, 5, 15 December 1953, carton 89, HJK Papers.

67. Mimeo, "Outline of Principles and Decisions By the Kaiser Foundation Trustees and Dr. Sidney R. Garfield," 9 October 1953, carton 89, HJK Papers.

68. Mimeo, "Remarks of Henry J. Kaiser to Be Given at Walnut Creek, 15 May 1953," carton 93, HJK Papers.

69. Collen, Bancroft ROHO history, 71. Kay describes this Medical Group decentralization plan in Kay, *Historical Review*, 81–82. The doctors were concerned not only about the fact that this would break down the collective power of the groups but that since their contract with the trustees of the Health Plan could be terminated by six months' notice on either side, the trustees might terminate a more expensive group in favor of a newer, less expensive one. See Thomas K. McCarthy to HJK, 11 November 1952, and attachment, "Description of Method of Operation of the Permanente Health Plan," carton 77, HJK Papers.

70. Trefethen, Bancroft ROHO history, 36.

71. George E. Link interview by Malca Chall, 1985, ibid., 32; Trefethen interview, ibid., 35.

72. Garfield interview by Stein, 30.
73. Memo, HJK to Dr. Wallace Neighbor, 16 September 1953, carton 91; HJK to Garfield, 14 October 1953, carton 89; HJK to Garfield, 12 November 1953, carton 92; file memorandum from HJK, 19 November 1953, carton 93, HJK Papers.
74. Collen, Bancroft ROHO history, 72.
75. Cutting, ibid., 51.
76. Memos, HJK to Trefethen, HJK to Garfield, 19 October 1953, carton 19, HJK Papers.

6   The Doctors' Revolt

1. Garfield interview by Foster. Kay interview by Foster.
2. Clifford H. Keene interview by author, 10 July 1986.
3. Ibid.
4. Ibid.
5. Keene, Bancroft ROHO history, 40–41.
6. Ibid.
7. Keene interview by author.
8. Keene, Bancroft ROHO history, 43.
9. Keene interview by author.
10. Garfield interview by Foster.
11. Both Ernest Saward and Keene remarked that Garfield did this. Saward, Bancroft ROHO history, 22; Keene interview by author.
12. Draft mimeo, Kaiser statement, 4 December 1953, carton 89, HJK Papers.
13. HJK to Garfield, 5 December 1953, carton 89, HJK Papers.
14. News release, 11 December 1953, ibid.; memo, "Miss Otto" to HJK, 14 December 1953; teletype, HJK to Keene, 15 December 1953, carton 99:22, EFK Papers.
15. HJK to Collen, 17 December 1953, carton 89, HJK Papers.
16. Keene, Bancroft ROHO history, 45.
17. Albert Deutsch, "Group Medicine: The Kaiser Health Plan," *Consumer Reports*, March 1957. The material for this article was gathered between 1952 and 1956. Corporate executives expressed concern that the Consumer's Union, which published the article, reached 600,000 subscribers heavily concentrated in "militant unions like those of CIO." Deutsch was described in a memo to Trefethen as "a reformer, liberal crusading writer," and the fear was expressed that he might be "unfriendly" to the Kaiser organization. See Robert C. Elliott to E. E. Trefethen, Jr., 7 August 1952, carton 77, and Hal Babbitt to Robert Elliott, 28 March 1956, carton 124, HJK Papers.
18. Mimeo, "Permanente Medical Group Members," 1955, carton 116, HJK Papers; Rothstein, *American Medical Schools*, 290 (table 15.4).
19. Friedman, Bancroft ROHO history, 54–55. These ideas are explored thoroughly in Regina Markell Morantz-Sanchez, *Sympathy and Science: Women Physicians in American Medicine* (New York: Oxford University Press, 1985), 3–7, 353–354.
20. Kay outlines these benefits in detail in Kay, *Historical Review*, 39–63.

21. Ibid., 108. In 1956 the doctor-member ratio was 1:1,229, with the goal to reduce that to 1:1,071, and ultimately to 1:1,000. This ratio was 1:944 by the mid-1970s. A favorable ratio was then relatively easy to maintain because the favorable atmosphere for HMO development greatly enhanced the Kaiser Permanente image as the model HMO. Also, elimination of the doctor's draft and growth of medical schools meant that the doctor shortage was becoming a surplus. The trend toward group practice in the 1970s marked a reversal in professional attitudes. Group physicians were only 1.2% of the medical profession in 1940; 2.6% in 1946; 5.2% in 1959; and 12.8% in 1969. By 1980, however, 25% of U.S. doctors practiced in groups. Also, between 1940 and 1950, the percentage of approved house staff positions hospitals were unable to fill rose from 10% to 30%. By 1957 hospitals needed over 12,000 interns a year, while medical schools were graduating less than 7,000 a year. For these statistics see Starr, *Social Transformation of American Medicine*, 425, 360.

22. Deutsch, "Group Medicine," 4.

23. Mimeo, Robert Elliott to EFK, "Highlights of Serious Deficit Trends of Hospitals," 13 February 1956, carton 132:2, EFK Papers.

24. Cutting, Bancroft ROHO history, 49; Collen, ibid., 74.

25. Evidence for this assumption is Keene's perception that Wallace Neighbor was the "ringleader" in the rebellion against Keene's appointment, and Cutting's remark that Baritell and Collen had strong disagreements in which Collen and Garfield were pitted against Baritell. Keene interview with author, 11 July 1986; Cutting, Bancroft ROHO, history, 49. While Cutting consistently expresses respect and admiration for Garfield's professional dedication, it appears that the experienced Dr. Cutting was able to walk a fine line between contending factions.

26. Collen, Bancroft ROHO history, 74–75.

27. Saward, ibid., 45.

28. Kay, *Historical Review*, 83.

29. Mimeo, "Relationship between the Kaiser Foundation and Permanente Physicians," c. 1 March 1955, carton 116, HJK Papers.

30. Quoted in Kay, *Historical Review*, 83; mimeo, "Draft of Minutes of Working Council," carton 116, HJK Papers.

31. Mimeo, "George Link's Legal Opinion Summarized," carton 116, HJK Papers.

32. Memo, Baritell, Collen, Cutting, Kay, Neighbor, Saward, Weiner to Edgar Kaiser, Trefethen, George Link, Garfield, Keene, 12 May 1955, ibid.

33. Ibid.

34. Link, Bancroft ROHO history, 23.

35. Ibid.

36. Draft of HJK letter that begins "Dear Doctor," 19 May 1955, carton 116, HJK Papers.

37. Ibid.

38. Mimeo, "Summary of Minutes of Working Council," 7, 21 June 1955, carton 116; mimeo, Kaiser statement, 6 June 1955, carton 117, HJK Papers. Kaiser had a detailed study made of the differences in revenue of a for-profit, physician-managed plan and of the established, tax-exempt "public trust." The figures favored the Kaiser Foundation structure: yearly "excess funds" generated by a nonprofit system were $60,000, by a tax-paying one, $5,000. Over a 20-year period almost $1.3 million more would be gained by the current Kaiser Foundation organization with doctors as contractors for a

percentage of income, than by the doctors if they attempted to create an independent organizational structure. See mimeo, "Salient Highlights of Weissman-Palmer Report," carton 117, HJK Papers.

39. Mimeo, "Salient Highlights."

40. Ibid.

41. "Summary of Minutes," 7, quoted in Kay, *Historical Review*, 83.

42. Collen, Bancroft ROHO history, 100.

43. "Summary of Minutes of Working Council," 7, 21 June 1955, carton 116, HJK Papers.

44. Cutting, Bancroft ROHO history, 61.

45. Participants in the Lake Tahoe meeting agree that Kaiser's emotionalism and personality made it impossible for him to negotiate with the doctors, and that he only attended one or two of the July meetings. Saward, Bancroft ROHO history, 88; Trefethen, Bancroft ROHO history, 43; Cutting, Bancroft ROHO history, 61. Trefethen quotation was made to Scott Fleming. Fleming, "Kaiser Permanente Overview," 29.

46. Trefethen, Bancroft ROHO history, 43; "Summary of Minutes of Working Council."

47. Link, Bancroft ROHO history, 35–36; Trefethen, Bancroft ROHO history, 42–43.

48. Kay interview by Foster.

49. Collen, Bancroft ROHO history, 82–84.

50. Kay, *Historical Review*, 154–155. Collen, Bancroft ROHO history, 83. Friedman, Bancroft ROHO history, 31.

51. Robert X. DeMangus, "We Take Issue with Dr. Alvarez," LACMA *Bulletin*, 14 July 1957, carton 193, HJK Papers.

52. Kay to Editor, LACMA *Bulletin*, 31 July 1957, carton 247, HJK Papers.

53. According to a Kaiser spokesperson, as late as 1981 the LACMA president published "an unfounded diatribe" against the Kaiser Permanente program. Fleming, *Kaiser-Permanente Program History*, 15.

54. Fleming, "Kaiser Permanente Overview," 33–34; Cutting, Bancroft ROHO history, 62.

55. Davis, *Medical Care for Tomorrow*, 230.

56. Fleming, "Kaiser Permanente Overview," 29–33; Kay, *Historical Review*, 85–98.

57. Link, Bancroft ROHO history, 36. Trefethen, ibid., 43.

58. Link, ibid., 36.

59. Keene letter to author, 22 July 1986; Keene interview by author, 11 July 1986.

60. Keene interview by author. Keene insists that he never had the title of medical director. His title was, in fact, unclear. He wrote to me, "Without and with various titles I was the fiscal manager of Kaiser Permanente from 1958 to 1975." Keene to author, 17 November 1989.

61. Wallace Croatman, "Are Labor Health Centers a Threat to Doctors?" *Medical Economics* 32 (October 1954), 112–113.

62. Starr, *Social Transformation of American Medicine*, 327–332.

63. William Issel, "Liberalism and Urban Policy in San Francisco From the 1930s to the 1960s," unpublished paper prepared for the 104th Annual Meeting of the American Historical Association, San Francisco, 28 December 1989; Garbarino, *Health Plans and Collective Bargaining*, 23–27.

64. Croatman, "Labor's Health Centers," 112–113.

65. Memo, Bob Elliott to HJK, 24 September 1954, attached to letter from the group suggesting the federation, carton 103, HJK Papers.

66. Handwritten memo, "C.K." to Bob Elliott, 18 June 1956; "Report of the President and Medical Director Ninth Annual Meeting of the Health Insurance Plan of Greater New York," 22 May 1956, carton 124, HJK Papers.

67. These events are summarized by Starr, *Social Transformation of American Medicine*, 327.

68. L. W. Larson, M.D., "Consumer-Sponsored Medical Care Plans From the Rural Perspective," n.d., and "Suggested Principles for Lay-Sponsored Voluntary Health Plans," Leonard W. Larson Papers, Box 1, Folder 21, University of North Dakota Library, Grand Forks, N.D.

69. Larson, "Consumer-Sponsored Medical Care Plans."

70. Report, *JAMA*, special edition, 17 January 1959, 12–18.

71. On the plans, ibid., 32, 78. On medical societies, ibid., 27.

72. Ibid., 92–93.

73. Keene letter to author, 22 July 1986; Keene interview by author, 11 July 1986.

74. Edith C. Bennett [HMSA Executive Secretary] to HJK, 23 January 1955; HJK to Hawaii Medical Association, 1 February 1955; HJK to Editor of the Hawaii Medical Journal, 23 April 1956, carton 193, HJK Papers.

75. Clippings, Henry J. Kaiser Hospitals—Hawaii Region Scrapbooks, vol 1., Bancroft Library, University of California, Berkeley, including: Charles Turner, "Kaiser Plans New $5,000,000 Hospital on Waikiki Beach; 15-Story Building, 192 Beds," *Hawaii's Territorial Newspaper*, 15 November 1955; "Kaiser Plans Skyscraper Hospital for Waikiki Area," *Honolulu Star-Bulletin*, 22 November 1955.

76. "Kaiser's Plan Still Alive," *Honolulu Star-Bulletin*, 22 November 1956; "Kaiser M.D. Finds Island Doctors Are Invited to Sign Up With Program," ibid., 25 April 1956; "Now Not Time to Build—Kaiser Leaves Hospital Issue Up to Physicians," *Honolulu Advisor*, 26 April 1956. Mimeo, "ILWU's English Language Program Digest . . . ," 8 February 1955, carton 193, HJK Papers.

77. Clipping, "Kaiser May Start Hospital Soon; Notes Attacks on Health Plan Dying Out," Hawaii Region Scrapbooks, vol. 2. Samuel L. Yee, M.D., HMA President, to HJK, 17 September 1957; HJK to Yee, 25 September 1957, carton 250, HJK Papers.

78. Editorial, "Kaiser Plan in Honolulu," *Hawaii Medical Journal*, July–August 1958, clipping, carton 250, HJK Papers; clipping, "Unionists May Be First Kaiser Clinic Patients; Rutledge, Tycoon Confer"; Tomi Kaizaw, "Kaiser Health Plan Is Assured Here; 5 Doctors Join," *Honolulu Star-Bulletin*, 22 May 1958, 1.

79. "Kaiser Health Plan Announcement Is Greeted With Mixed Reactions," *Honolulu Star-Bulletin*, 22 May 1958, 1, Hawaii Region Scrapbooks, vol. 2.

80. Fleming, "Kaiser Permanente Overview," 36–37.

81. Ibid.

82. Press release, Kaiser Foundation Health Plan, 26 August 1960, carton 251, HJK Papers.

83. Ibid.; press release, Kaiser Foundation Medical Center, 27 August 1960, carton 251, HJK Papers.

84. Memo, Henry J. Kaiser to Sidney R. Garfield, with copy to Mrs. Henry J. Kaiser, 28 January 1955, carton 117, HJK Papers.

85. HJK to E. E. Trefethen, Jr., 19 August 1961, carton 255, HJK Papers.

86. Keene, telephone conversation and correspondence with the author, 11, 17 November 1989.

Conclusion

1. U.S. Department of Health and Human Services, Public Health Service, National Center for Health Statistics, *United States Health and Prevention Profile* (Hyattsville, Md.: U.S. Government Printing Office, 1983), 177, 184–185.

2. Starr, *Social Transformation of American Medicine*; Grant, "California's Health Care Marketplace"; Stevens, *In Sickness and In Wealth*, 301–302.

3. These ideas are partly derived from: Parsons, "Social Change and Medical Organization," 21–33; Hyde and Wolff, "American Medical Association," 975–1022; Burnham, "American Medicine's Golden Age," 1474–1479.

4. Although 71% of the more than 363,000 federal employees who chose to enroll in group practice plans joined Kaiser, about 4.7 million joined Blue Cross–Blue Shield and 1.5 million the Aetna Life and Casualty indemnity plan. Yet federal employees made up 14% of total Kaiser subscribers by 1969. Nygren and Childs, *Federal Employees' Health Benefits Program*, 7–11.

5. Garbarino, *Health Plans and Collective Bargaining*, 100–101. Labor economist Garbarino makes the assessment of the status of Kaiser Permanente and its receding threat to organized medicine in the late 1950s. By the 1970s, however, Kaiser penetration had increased to as high as 29% at Richmond. Somers, *Kaiser-Permanente Medical Care Program*, 198 (table 3).

6. Mimeo, Walter Phair to HJK, excerpts from "President's Commission on Building America's Health," 27 March 1953, carton 88, HJK Papers.

7. Starr, *Social Transformation of American Medicine*, 309–310, 331–332. For details on income and insurance rates, see Starr, pp. 309–310.

8. Table, "Kaiser Foundation Health Plan Membership As At December 31st For The Years 1950 to 1963," carton 247, HJK Papers.

9. Peter Grant documents this strategy among the county and state medical societies in Washington, Oregon, and California in Grant, "California's Health Care Marketplace," 72. Overwhelmed by consumer demand in 1989, Permanente hired 400 new physicians in the region and more than 400 the following year. Despite a 19.6% rate increase for 1990, the highest since 1952 and the first large expansion program, and 18% for 1991, Kaiser still cost 30% to 50% less than most indemnity plans, and 10% to 20% less than other HMOs. Nationwide membership grew 9.6% a year by decade's end and will end the twentieth century with a ten-year $8.6 billion capital spending plan in California, and a $3.6 billion five-year expansion in northern California. Russell, "Kaiser's Rates to Climb 19%" and "Kaiser Rate Rises Amid HMO Turmoil."

10. *Statistical Trends; A Demographic, Utilization, and Financial Summary* (Oakland: Kaiser Permanente Medical Care Program, 1990), 5, 10.

11. These studies include Starr, *Social Transformation of American Medicine*; Fox, *Health Policies, Health Politics*, 47–48; Stevens, *In Sickness and In Wealth*.

12. Fox, *Health Policies, Health Politics*, 47–48.

13. Roy Porter, "The Gift Relation: Philanthropy and Provincial Hospitals in Eighteenth-century England," in Lindsay Granshaw and Roy Porter, eds., *The Hospital in History* (London: Routlege, 1989). For this description of the paradox embodied in the U.S. hospital system: Stevens, *In Sickness and in Wealth*. For earlier applications of traditional paternalistic and community concepts in the U.S. hospital see Rosenberg, *The Care of Strangers*; for case studies, Diana Elizabeth Long and Janet Golden, eds., *The American General Hospital: Communities and Social Contexts* (Ithaca, N.Y.: Cornell University Press, 1989).

14. An extreme form of this reduction of human life to material terms is shown in a recent article that itemizes Washington's price tag for the "cost-benefit" of the human body. The U.S. Consumer Product Safety Commission values it at $2 million; the Environmental Protection Agency at $8 million; and the Nuclear Regulatory Commission at $5 million. Christopher Scanlan, "Putting a Price Tag on Life—U.S. weighs costs, benefits of tax dollars," *Marin Independent Journal*, 26 August 1990, F6.

15. For the role of the social sciences in U.S. universities before World War II, and the discrediting of the belief that there were discoverable, immutable scientific laws governing society in the irresolution of the nature-nurture controversy, Hamilton Cravens, *The Triumph of Evolution: The Heredity-Environment Controversy, 1900–1941*, 2d ed. (Baltimore: Johns Hopkins University Press, 1988), 135, 211. For the academic discipline of "social medicine" in the European and U.S. context, I have drawn on Porter and Porter, "What Was Social Medicine?"

16. *Historical Statistics*, 75; Starr, *Social Transformation of American Medicine*, 425; Stevens, *In Sickness and in Wealth*, 403n46.

17. E. Richard Weinerman, "Patients' Perceptions of Group Medical Care, Review and Analysis of Studies on Choice and Utilization of Prepayment Group Practice Plans," *American Journal of Public Health* 54 (1964), 881–882.

18. Wallace H. Cook, "Profile of the Permanente Physician," in Somers, *Kaiser-Permanente Medical Care Program*, 104; National Advisory Commission on Health Manpower, *The Kaiser Foundation Medical Care Program*, vol. 11 (Washington, D.C.: U.S. Government Printing Office, 1967), 198–199 [hereafter NACHM Report]; mimeo, "Magnitude of Physician Top Management Responsibilities . . . Selection System to Find Doctors of Teamwork Temperaments and Professionally Qualified for Group Practice," 6 December 1955, carton 309, HJK Papers.

19. National Advisory Commission on Health Manpower, 206. Nygren and Childs, *Federal Employees' Health Benefits Program*, 6–9.

20. Rothstein, *American Medical Schools*, 212–213.

21. Study cited in Stevens, *In Sickness and in Wealth*, 405n22; cf. *Medical Care Program for Steelworkers and Their Families* (Pittsburgh: United Steelworkers of America, 1960), tables 34, 35.

22. Annual admissions per 1,000 were 80 in 1965, down from 88 in 1960; nationally they were 138, up from 129 in 1960. Annual per person hospital expenses rose 15.4% at Kaiser (to almost $30), but 49.7% nationally (to almost $50). Reduced hospitalization produced a substantial savings in

Kaiser Permanente operation, making the annual per patient cost up to 45% less than the medical expense of average Californians. NACHM Report, 206.

23. This framework for chronological stages is applied to the HMO movement as a whole in Merwyn R. Greenlick, Donald K. Freeborn, and Clyde R. Pope, eds., *Health Care Research in an HMO—Two Decades of Discovery* (Baltimore: Johns Hopkins University Press, 1988), 3–10.

24. Table, "Health Plan Membership for Selected Years," carton 339, HJK Papers; Fleming, "Kaiser-Permanente Program History," 29–32; Kaiser Permanente Medical Care Program, *Facts 1990*, 1; NACHM report, 192, 201; Russell, "Kaiser Rate Rises Amid HMO Turmoil."

25. Health Policy Advisory Center, Editorial, "The Kaiser Plan," *Health/Pac Bulletin* 55 (November 1973), 1.

26. Starr, *Social Transformation of American Medicine*, 396–397; Stevens, *In Sickness and In Wealth*, 302–303.

Index